W9-CAI-000

MASSAGE
FOR TOTAL
STRESS RELIEF

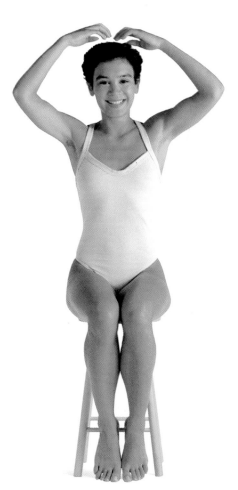

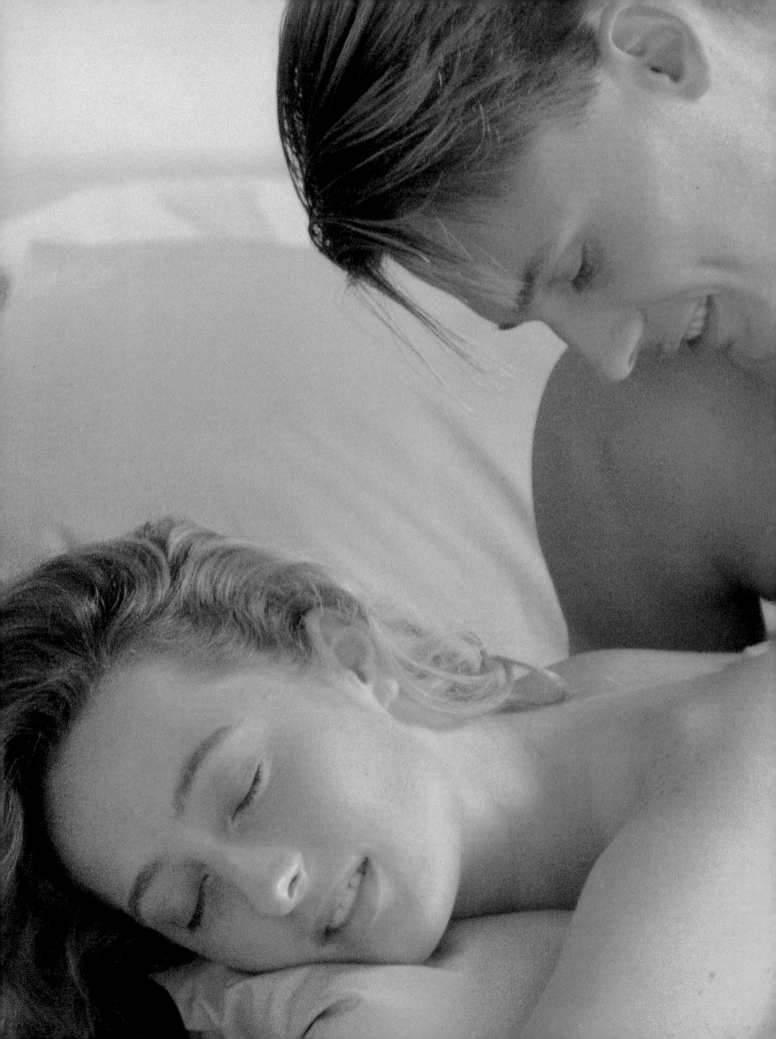

MASSAGE
FOR TOTAL
STRESS RELIEF

NITYA LACROIX

RANDOM HOUSE
NEW YORK

[DK]

A DORLING KINDERSLEY BOOK

*To Rachel French, with so much
gratitude and thanks for your
fantastic support this year*

Art Editor
Tina Vaughan

Project Editor
Susannah Marriott

Managing Editor
Daphne Razazan

Managing Art Editor
Anne-Marie Bulat

Copyright © 1990 Dorling Kindersley Limited, London
Text copyright © 1990 by Nitya Lacroix

All rights reserved under International
and Pan-American Copyright Conventions.
Published in the United States by
Random House, Inc., New York.

Library of Congress Cataloguing-in-Publication Data
Lacroix, Nitya.
    Massage for total stress relief / by Nitya Lacroix.
    p. cm.
    ISBN 0-679-73511-9
    1. Massage. 2. Relaxation. 3. Typology (Psychology). I. Title.
RA780.5.L32 1991 616.8'22--dc20 90-49648

Manufactured in the United States of America
98765432   24689753   23456789
First US Edition

CONTENTS

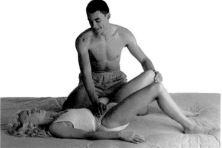

INTRODUCTION

Stress. It takes its toll on our bodies, minds and emotions. We feel it in tight muscles and a clenched jaw, in nagging fatigue and sharp mood swings. We feel cut off from ourselves and the world around us. In this time of increasing pressures, where personal and global tensions affect our daily lives, stress is inevitable - and the ability to relax is essential. When relaxed, you feel whole and at ease with yourself and your surroundings. This sense of harmony within body, mind and emotions provides a deep nourishment which replenishes your resources, restores your vitality, and lets you enjoy life fully.

This book focuses on massage as a medium for stress relief and relaxation. It shows you how to identify your own physical tension patterns, and explains their relationship with your underlying emotions. It also helps you to understand what causes you stress as an individual. Once you have understood your stress patterns, the book leads you on to methods for relaxation. As well as massage, it offers simple self-help techniques, such as movement, meditation, body and breath awareness, and exercises that correctly align the body. It will also help you to recognize where and why tension is held in a friend, colleague, or partner's body, and show you how together to release that tension, restore relaxation and boost vitality. Massage is an experience to share, and I hope this book will help you enjoy the satisfaction of both giving and receiving massages.

Massage for Total Stress Relief is based on the intrinsic relationship of the body, mind, emotions and spirit that makes every one of us a unique and whole person. Each of these aspects affects the other, and health and happiness result from achieving harmony and balance between all these parts. Massage is one of the most effective and beneficial ways to reach and relax the whole person.

THE ANCIENT ROOTS OF MASSAGE

Massage is an ancient science and art. From the beginning of time, men and women have intuitively known that touch and the laying of hands on the body can evoke profound changes in body and mind. It is natural to reach out and touch. We do so as a means of comfort and communication, and in order to share love and affection. We instinctively rub and soothe painful parts of the body, and caress or hold someone in a gesture of sympathy and concern. Historical records show that massage has been valued for thousands of years and in many different civilizations because of its healing power, its ability to restore good humor, to rid the body of pain, to rejuvenate tired and tense muscles, and to boost energy. Long before people became dependent on medical drugs and highly sophisticated technology to fight disease, massage was applied, often together with herbs and natural potions, to combat physical and mental ailments.

Massage and touch mean different things to different cultures. In many Eastern countries families massage each other regularly. While any display of sexual affection within these societies is strictly taboo, they are aware of the far-reaching benefits of massage and are not afraid to rub each others' limbs to ease away tension and relieve pain. In the West, where sexuality has become almost a media commodity, we have become frightened of touching each other outside the safety of an intimate relationship. It is because we are so deprived of spontaneous affection and touch that massage plays such an essential role, allowing us to receive the vital nourishment that a comforting touch imparts. Combined with the right techniques, and a caring and sympathetic attitude, massage is one of the most healing, deeply relaxing experiences there is. When receiving a massage, we become open, responsive and whole. When giving a massage, we express ourselves and show care through our hands. Massage is a creative art through which both giver and receiver explore and discover themselves.

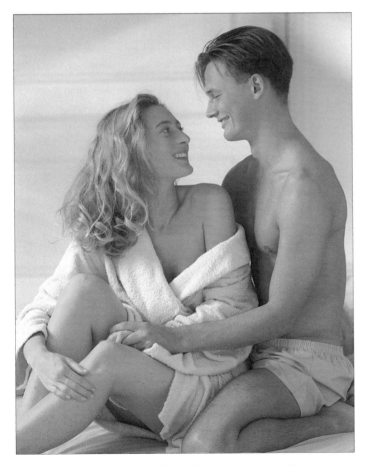

Relaxation and vitality allow you to rediscover joy and playfulness, intensifying your pleasure in life and relationships.

THE BENEFITS OF MASSAGE

Throughout my many years' experience as a massage therapist and as a teacher, I have worked with people of varying body types, characters and types of emotional behavior. It has always amazed me how diverse the health-giving effects of massage can be. In its most simple form, massage is a curative treatment for the muscles and the body's soft tissue. Stroking, rubbing and kneading the body all relieve tension from and restore suppleness to tight and sore muscles. These tactile actions improve blood circulation and so help the cardiovascular system carry oxygen and nutrients to cells, tissue, and the internal organs. The strokes also break down waste products trapped in muscles, assisting decongestion and elimination, while they boost the body's lymphatic system in its vital cleansing role. The friction of hands on the skin, often called the body's largest organ, directly affects the nervous system, which carries messages from the brain to all parts of the body via the spinal cord. Depending on the type of strokes used, massage stimulates or soothes this system of nerve responses. In these ways, massage can be both relaxing and invigorating, and these physical results alone induce a state of relief and well-being.

THE STRESS RESPONSE

Stress, to some degree, is an essential part of life. It motivates us and provides the impetus to be creative, meet challenges, change our circumstances, take risks and act positively. Without stress in our lives, we would become unhealthily passive and inert, unable to initiate or respond to events. However, in serious instances stress can lead to a range of illnesses, including high blood pressure, coronary disease, ulcers, digestive disorders, exhaustion, insomnia, depression, lowered immune resistance, and emotional break-down. Even short-term stress can affect the body detrimentally, causing painful muscles, headaches and back trouble.

Whether real or imagined, life-threatening or a common occurrence, whether physical, mental, or emotional, stress stimulates the nervous system. It triggers an involuntary response and creates biochemical changes in the body which cause stress hormones such as adrenalin to flood to the organs. Changes follow: the heart rate speeds up, oxygen intake increases, blood pressure rises, the digestive system closes down, muscles tense and the body sweats. These changes prepare the body to react to stress in an appropriate way — a "fight or flight" response. Years ago, this response could have made the difference between living and dying. In the face of danger the choice was to confront it or flee, and in either action the charge of energy built up in the body was released.

The tensions that surround us in the modern world are now more insidious. The pressure to succeed, the bombardment of sensations, family breakdown, loneliness and isolation, financial worries, and the constant change of society's structures cause these age-old stress responses in the body. Yet our ability to express and then discharge tension is now more curtailed. If we feel unable to control a situation, or even to pinpoint the stress factor, if the tension is prolonged or not discharged in an appropriate way, then the pent-up nervous energy will deplete our natural resources and erode our health and mental well-being.

AN ANTIDOTE TO STRESS

Although our physical responses to stress are involuntary, we can control the balance between activity and relaxation in our lives and so replenish the energy we use up with day to day tensions. If we understand who we are as individuals, we will be better able to gauge our responses, our capabilities and our vulnerabilities. By learning to recognize those situations that cause us undue stress, we can make conscious choices about our lives. While a certain amount of stress is unavoidable, we need to tend and care for ourselves as we might care for others. If we recognize our body's tension signs, we can discharge that energy by moving, exercising and dancing, and by communicating with people we trust. We can learn to control the body's stress response by relaxing, breathing deeply, meditating, and by developing awareness of the mind and body.

Massage is a welcome antidote to stress and the destructive accumulative effects on the body of stress-related illness. It is the perfect way to regain a holistic balance and break free from the grip of tension. There are few other opportunities in life where all one has to do is to receive, be touched and cared for. Massage creates precious time for the body and mind to relax and switch off from the hectic whirl of life. In doing so, energy spent in dealing with stress is replenished, and the body's innate healing process is set in motion. This message of restoration is sent through the entire nervous network of the body: beneficial change is brought to the vital organs, the mind is calmed, the emotions are settled, and our sense of wholeness is restored.

MASSAGE AND EMOTIONAL TENSION

In *Massage for Total Stress Relief*, I have tried to sketch out the relationship between character, emotions and muscular tension, and its effects on the body and posture. This concept was understood by ancient Eastern cultures, especially the Mongolian samurai, who also recognized the psychosomatic benefits of massage. Before battle, a soldier would apply strong massage to his body to rid it of the memories of fear and pain which he believed lay trapped in his muscles and would inhibit his bravery and courage. The warrior understood a concept of "protective armor" in the body. He knew that when the muscles tighten against the experience of a painful emotion or physical trauma, the memory of this is held within the tissue and then continues to affect the behavior, the psyche, and eventually the whole structure of the body.

In the first half of this century Wilhelm Reich, psychiatrist and disciple of Sigmund Freud, declared that by releasing the body's tension, or "character armor", one could heal psychological and emotional problems. In the last decades this alternative approach to healing, which encompasses the relationship of the body, the mind and the emotions, has become more accepted in the West. The body is perceived as an open map on which one's life history is charted. Our childhood experiences, relationships, thoughts and feelings, hopes and fears, emotional behavior and character are, in this holistic concept, constantly broadcast by the body in the way we move and use our muscles, and in the way we breathe and stand.

Massage for Total Stress Relief makes no pretence at covering the enormity of this subject, and readers who would like to investigate these concepts further should turn to the bibliography. Instead, this book introduces the basic ideas of how the body reflects who we are, the causes of stress and tension, and how, through touch, awareness and massage, we can relax body and mind, and explore the interplay between them. This book, I hope, will be the beginning of an exciting journey of discovery.

TOTAL RELAXATION

A massage integrates the body, mind and underlying emotions in subtle ways. It does not directly confront tension, but seduces the muscles and tissue into deep relaxation. When massage is given with care and full attention, and with a loving quality of touch, the effects can go much deeper than the body and reach the inner recesses of the mind and emotions. Massage instigates the process of relaxation and inner harmony. It helps the body to heal itself. Yet the most profound experiences of massage come in those special moments when you or your partner feels renewed, whole and in balance. At these times it is possible to feel that it is no longer the body being touched, but the very core, the essential self. It is here that the doing stops and the being exists without stress or tension. I believe that within all of us, beyond our character, our psychology and our physical anatomy, flows a pure and unimpeded river of life energy. Within an atmosphere of love and trust, massage and touch, even in their simplest form, can take you to its source. It is at this source that we can exist in a state of total relaxation.

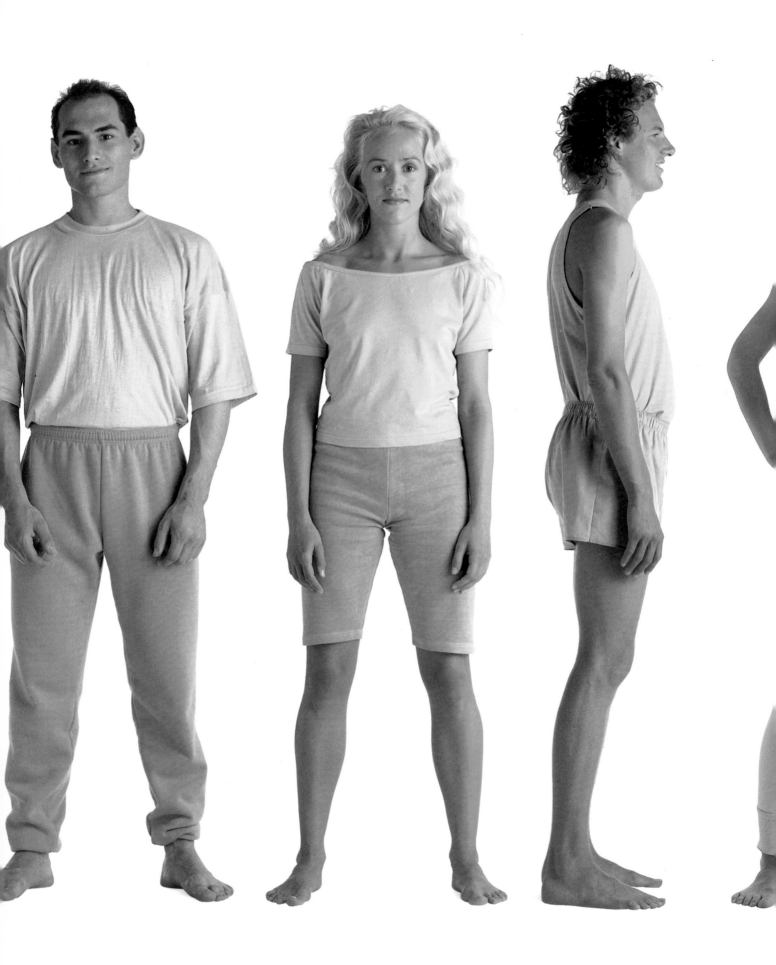

1
BODY PROFILES

Learning to understand your body is the key to unlocking tension and enjoying a deep sense of relaxation. By showing how to identify your own physical and emotional body type, this section helps you to discover the causes of tension, and pinpoint where and how it affects your body.

KEY TENSION AREAS
WHERE · AND · HOW · STRESS · AFFECTS · THE · BODY

Tension forms in the body as a protection against physical and emotional trauma. It tends to root itself between the major body parts, creating tight bands of muscles that cause one area of the body to be cut off physically and emotionally from another. Thus, stored and chronic tension can fragment the wholeness and unity of the body, isolate the mind from its intrinsic responses and feelings, and numb and suppress the emotions. It has always been intuitively understood that stress and tension affect the body. Whether you "carry the world on your shoulders" when burdened, have "butterflies in the stomach" when anxious or excited, "grit your teeth," show "backbone," or "go weak at the knees" when confronted with crisis, language richly describes the effects of such trauma on key areas of the body.

THE BACK

Acting as a protective shell to the body, the back stores feelings of anger and fear as it tightens against everyday stress. It is one of the most common areas of tension and pain. Harmful posture habits can result in over-extended or contracted muscles along the spine and in the lower back.

EASING THE BACK
- *Spine and lower back* pages 108–109.
- *The guard* pages 48–49.
- *The stoic* pages 78–79.
- *The victim* pages 54–55.

The face tenses as you try to mask your emotions

The shoulders clearly indicate your physical, mental and emotional well-being

The solar plexus, a nerve complex behind the stomach, can pulsate with pent-up feelings of fear, anxiety and anger

The pelvic area is linked with emotions concerning survival, anger, sexuality and pleasure

THE FACE

Nowhere are you more likely to reveal your most private thoughts, feelings and responses than in the face. The facial muscles tense in order to hide vulnerability and present an "acceptable" mask to the world. Key points of tension are the mouth, jaw, and around the eyes.

EASING THE FACE
- *Head and face* pages 106-107.
- *Executive stress* pages 86-87.

A key area for relaxed and easy posture, the knees also reveal attitudes toward control, fear and weakness

The legs relate to childhood emotions and attitudes such as rage and stubbornness

The feet can be a guide to your physical and emotional stability

NECK AND SHOULDERS

We all experience tension in this area at some time. The shoulders are a buffer between mind and body and tighten to restrain uncomfortable emotions. Attitudes toward work and responsibility are reflected here. When relaxed, the shoulders and neck are vital for a balanced body.

EASING NECK AND SHOULDERS
- *Neck and shoulders* pages 103-105.
- *Roots and wings* pages 40-41.
- *Sedentary stress* pages 90-91.

ABDOMEN AND DIAPHRAGM

The abdomen tightens to suppress strong "gut-level" emotions. A tense diaphragm, a large muscle separating abdomen and chest, will divide the body. This blocks the flow of breath, reduces energy, and separates the instinctive emotions from the more vulnerable feelings in the chest.

EASING ABDOMEN AND DIAPHRAGM
- *The superman* pages 72-77.
- *The intellectual* page 68.

THE PELVIS

The pelvic area supports the vital organs and upper body. Postural tension can pull the pelvis out of correct alignment, making it slump forward or lock back. This strains the lower back and abdominal muscles. The position and tension of the pelvic area reveals attitudes toward sexuality, pleasure, and life itself.

EASING THE PELVIS
- *Pelvis and groin* page 102.
- *Sensual strokes* pages 116-17.

LEGS AND KNEES

This area reveals the "stand" you take in the world, and so reflects self-image. Rigid legs are an unstable foundation and indicate emotional insecurity. The knees manifest feelings toward fear and control, submission and weakness.

EASING LEGS AND KNEES
- *Legs and knees* pages 100-101.
- *The warrior* page 62.
- *The stoic* pages 80-81.

FEET AND ANKLES

How the feet are used and how much contact they make with the ground is often indicative of how you cope with reality. Unevenly distributed weight can cause tension in the feet and ankle joints, affecting ease of movement.

EASING FEET AND ANKLES
- *Feet and ankles* pages 98-99.
- *The stoic* pages 82-83.
- *Self-massage* page 94.

STRESS & YOUR BODY
YOUR · POSTURE · AND · HOW · TO · IDENTIFY · YOUR · BODY · PROFILE

Your body constantly mirrors every aspect of yourself. Your personality, underlying emotions, attitudes, and how you relate to the world and others - all are apparent in your body. How you think and feel defines not only the way you stand and move, it determines the ease of your muscles, the areas in which you feel tension, and your breathing patterns. In addition, the body is affected by everyday situations that create stress, causing the muscles to tighten, and the flow of breath to diminish. Whether tension is emotional or physical, chronic or acute, it affects health and happiness, and is obvious in your posture and the way you move.

PERSONALITY AND POSTURE

When we are small babies, our bodies and emotions are at their most spontaneous and vibrant. We sleep when tired, play when happy and contented, cry when frustrated, eat when hungry, and exhibit fierce anger when our needs are unmet. Our feelings are constantly expressed and released through the body, and when we receive outside stimulus, be it through food or touch, our sense of well-being is nourished. We are at one with ourselves and the environment. As we grow, we begin to perceive ourselves as separate from the surroundings and family we depend on for survival. We struggle to adapt to and survive the ever-increasing demands made upon us. We learn how to behave, and how to win approval and love, by controlling our urges and behavior to suit others. Physically, we repress emotions and spontaneous vitality by diminishing breathing and contracting the muscles, and this habit becomes a chronic, unconscious pattern that affects every aspect of our lives. Muscles and posture develop according to

the evolving personality. As tension and stress increases, we cut ourselves off from our true feelings and innate responses. We develop fixed attitudes about ourselves and the world which affect our relationships, ease of motion, and the entire balance and posture of the body.

Other factors affect the body as we develop. Adolescents may be influenced by current media heroes: the couldn't-care-less slump of a pop idol, the superhero's macho posture, the catwalk model's backward-tilted glide, or the sex siren's chest out and buttocks back pose. If such images become a fixed posture in our own bodies, the results are disastrous.

THE EFFECTS OF GRAVITY

Thousands of years ago, the human species did something extraordinary: it stood up against the weight and pull of gravity. Even now, the body has not fully adjusted to this major step in our evolution. The pull that gravity exerts is a heavy toll on our upright posture. This is exhibited by the tension often felt in our most basic actions, such as walking, sitting and standing. Whenever there is an imbalance in its structure, the body struggles to compensate. For instance, if the head leans forward, the pelvis and knees may lock back to prevent you from falling over. A twist in the shoulder can cause the opposing hip to rotate in the opposite direction. All this creates muscular tension in the body as the muscles take over the work of the skeletal system, which is designed to carry our weight. Emotional patterns and ingrained attitudes may dictate whether your particular body type will tense and fight against the effects of gravity, or collapse under it in defeat.

THE BODY PROFILES

This section of the book features a series of familiar body profiles which demonstrates the relationship between emotions, self-image, attitudes, and posture. These profiles are a generalization of common body shapes and emotional patterns. It may be possible to recognize your own tension patterns in them, and through this to understand how and where stress affects your body. The profiles are followed by massage programs designed to work on the tension patterns associated with particular body types.

As you respond emotionally and physically to different phases of your life, you may be able to recognize yourself in several of the body types. Or you may identify with one body profile and recognize a similarity in attitude. Yet it is important not to identify wholly with one profile: we are all complex in our make-up, and essentially each of us is individual, unique, and capable of change.

HOW TO IDENTIFY YOUR PROFILE

To begin to recognize your body profile, or aspects of it, take into consideration your attitudes, values, ambitions, fears, and career choices. Carefully examine your emotional behavior and look at which feelings you most identify with. Ask yourself a number of key questions. What role do you play in relationships? How do you react to stressful situations? What is your self-image? Locate the areas in your body in which you feel any tension or discomfort, and use the body awareness exercise on pages 16-17. Look at yourself in a mirror and assess your posture. Now compare these findings with the body profiles shown on pages 18-29.

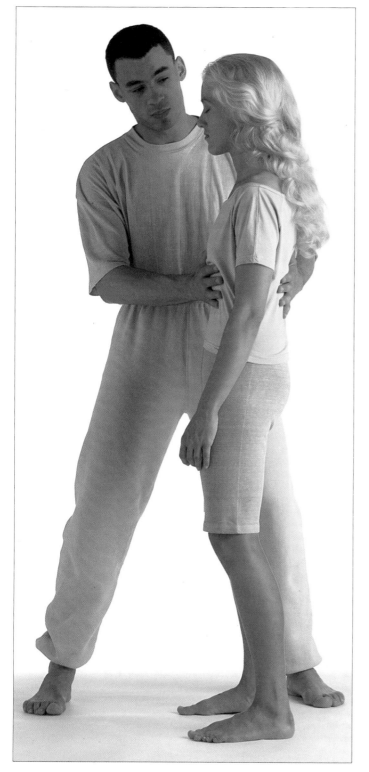

Discovering your body type, its tension patterns and ways to achieve relaxation is an experience which can be shared with partners and friends.

WHICH BODY TYPE ARE YOU?

The following information is a quick reference guide to the body type profiles that follow. The descriptions will help you to recognize your body type or types by identifying key characteristics, including attitude, responses, emotional make-up, and image.

The guard pages 18-19
This is the most generic of all the body types, and a common tension pattern for many people when under stress. Key characteristics: defensive, tight, contracted, cautious, frozen, woundup, tense.

The victim pages 20-21
Both the body and character of this body type show tendencies to collapse when faced with pressure. Key characteristics: insecure, unassertive, weak, dependent, sociable, sad, a sense of failure.

The warrior pages 22-23
This type is rigid and inflexible in both body and character. Key characteristics: assertive, a fighter, responsible, protective, ambitious, prone to anger, a leader.

The intellectual pages 24-25
Often contracted and uncoordinated physically, this body type has well-developed mental capabilities. Key characteristics: disconnected, withdrawn, remote, fearful, intelligent, imaginative, academic, feelings of isolation.

The superman pages 26-27
This body type often has a dominating personality. Key characteristics: self-important, must be the center of attention, aggressive, charming, controlling, persuasive.

The stoic pages 28-29
This body type is often burdened and heavy-looking and may have a strong tendency to endure. Key characteristics: reliable, resentful, stubborn, self-sacrificing, loyal, a sense of being stuck.

IDENTIFYING YOUR TENSION PATTERNS

WE ALL KNOW WHAT OUR BODIES look like, and the image we present to the world, but it is important to listen to what the body is saying to us internally. To initiate relaxation and beneficial changes, we need to find our stress patterns and learn where and why tension forms in the muscles, joints, and body alignment. This exercise helps lead toward a deeper understanding of your body: its areas of tension and ease, breathing patterns and underlying emotions. Becoming aware of your stress patterns may be a shock, but recognizing them without judgment is the first step in freeing and relaxing the whole body.

1 Stand as you do normally. Do not arrange your body in a "correct" posture.

2 Close your eyes and imagine you have internal eyes focusing on your body. Carefully pass over each part of it, moving up from the toes. Pay special attention to the body's key tension areas (see pages 12-13).

3 Ask yourself the following questions about each area of your body:

"Does it feel loose and relaxed, or tense and tight?"
"Am I comfortable or does standing strain this area?"
"Do I feel collapsed and contracted, or expanded and aligned here?"
"Does this area feel alive, or tense and dead?"
"Is this part of my body in balance, or does it rotate and tilt?"
"Am I breathing fully or shallowly, and is my breath reaching this part of my body?"
"Does this area feel vulnerable, open and relaxed, or is it tense and like armor?"

4 Then focus on areas of the body that are crucial for a relaxed and balanced posture. ▷

Are your neck and head in line with the spine, stretched forward, or compressed back? Does your neck release upward from the shoulders?

Is your spine rigid, collapsed, tense and tight, or lengthened and light?

Does your pelvis support your torso, or is it locked back or slumped under?

Are your knees flexible and loose, or locked back tightly?

Are your ankles tight and strained? Do they support your weight evenly, collapse inward or tip outward?

Do your feet support your weight evenly? Do you lean forward or backward over them? Do they feel stable on the ground?

Is your jaw tight and stressed, or loose and relaxed? Does it jut forward or pull back?

Is your head heavy or light? Does it feel glued to your neck or is there a feeling of space between the head and neck?

How fully do you breathe into your chest? Do your lungs expand up to your shoulders when you inhale? Does your chest feel open and relaxed, or heavily protected?

Does your stomach feel tense or relaxed? Is your breath reaching down into the lower abdomen?

5 Now shake your body from top to toe for several minutes to release all the tensions you have observed. Focus especially on the tense areas. Breathe deeply as you shake, let go of your body completely, and make sounds.

6 Stop shaking and stand still. Feel the blood pulsing through your veins, your heart beating vibrantly, and your deepened breathing. Now sit or lie down, and allow your body to relax totally.

17

THE GUARD
A · DEFENSIVE · BODY · AND · HOW · TO · RELAX · IT

To some degree it is natural to turn one's body into a safe shell for protection, and retreat beneath it when faced with stress. Some people, however, constantly create this defensive armor: tightening the muscles and restricting breathing to control uncomfortable feelings and guard against stress. The *guard type* lives in a state of tension, and rather than responding spontaneously to events, often anticipates a crisis from past memories or anxiety about the future. Tension builds up but fails to be released when the trauma passes. Eventually this tension reaches a breaking point, and even a minor incident can cause an outburst of emotion.

CHARACTERISTICS

The *guard type* personality tends to hold his breath or breathe shallowly. There is an underlying sense of control and defensiveness, and the response to stress is often one of contraction which may be reflected in a "frozen" posture. This person can convey the impression of a tightly wound up coil, ready to spring into action, and when this becomes habitual, the predominant tension areas are the upper back, shoulders, neck, chest, and diaphragm.

SIGNS OF STRESS

■ Face muscles tighten.
■ Shoulders rise up in defence or round over to protect the heart area, the site of vulnerable feelings.
■ Tension in the back, shoulders, and neck will cause pain.
■ The rib cage and back pull upward, reducing the flow of breath through the abdomen.
■ Joints become constricted as physical and emotional energy is contracted.

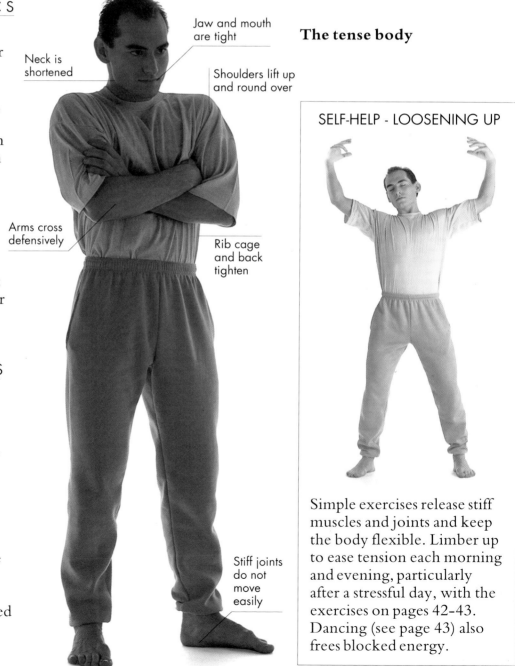

Jaw and mouth are tight

Neck is shortened

Shoulders lift up and round over

The tense body

Arms cross defensively

Rib cage and back tighten

Stiff joints do not move easily

SELF-HELP · LOOSENING UP

Simple exercises release stiff muscles and joints and keep the body flexible. Limber up to ease tension each morning and evening, particularly after a stressful day, with the exercises on pages 42–43. Dancing (see page 43) also frees blocked energy.

RELAXATION PROGRAM
PAGES 46-49

MASSAGING THE CHEST MUSCLES, back, shoulders, and neck relieves tension and pain in the upper body.

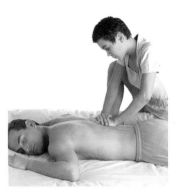

Back Stretching strokes over the back will free tension in the muscles that support the spine.

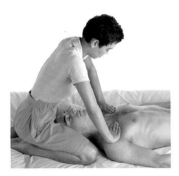

Chest Strokes on the muscles of the upper chest will bring width and release to the area.

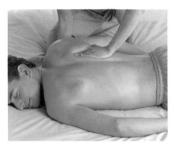

Shoulder blades Loosening tight muscles encourages the shoulder blades to relax.

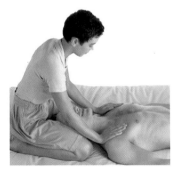

Shoulders Tight and tense shoulders benefit from this rhythmic, rocking movement that relaxes the shoulders.

The open body

FURTHER RELAXATION

■ Lift and release the joints and limbs. See *the warrior* pages 58–63.
■ Ease the face. See *head and face* pages 106–107.
■ Massage tight neck muscles. See *shoulders and neck* pages 103–105.
■ Relax the diaphragm and abdomen. See *the superman* pages 72–77.
■ Free the lower body. See *feet and ankles*; *legs and knees* pages 98–101.

THE VICTIM
A · COLLAPSED · BODY · AND · HOW · TO · RELAX · IT

To function well when faced with challenges you need to be able to stand up for yourself, and feel independent and secure. Without these qualities people may feel like the victims of circumstance. Under stress, and unable to take charge, they are likely to collapse both physically and emotionally. When this attitude is deep-rooted, the posture slumps downward as if the body cannot withstand the pull of gravity or the strains of tension. This stooped posture reveals an inner sense of inadequacy or helplessness, and an underlying dependency on others. The basic response to stress of the *victim type* is one of flight or giving up.

CHARACTERISTICS

Energy is low and the body tends to look weak. The posture reflects this person's inner feelings of collapse and helplessness. Someone with *victim type* tendencies may feel unable to take control of life. The *victim type* finds it easy to express vulnerable emotions, but being assertive, or exposing more hidden feelings such as resentment and anger, is much more difficult.

SIGNS OF STRESS

■ The skin is often pale and the muscles are undertoned. This is linked with the lack of breath taken into the body, which prevents the circulatory system from nourishing the body's vital organs fully.
■ The arms and hands hang limply from the shoulders. This reflects an inability to "reach out" to others.
■ The head tends to drop forward, putting strain on the neck and shoulders and contracting the throat.
■ The shoulders slump.
■ The chest is collapsed and hollow.

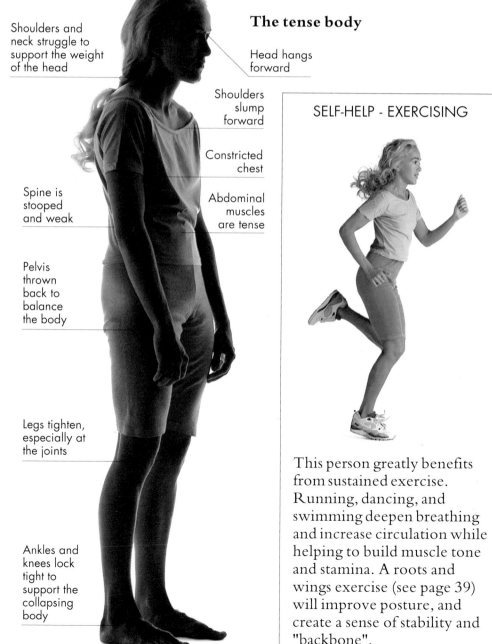

Shoulders and neck struggle to support the weight of the head

Spine is stooped and weak

Pelvis thrown back to balance the body

Legs tighten, especially at the joints

Ankles and knees lock tight to support the collapsing body

The tense body

Head hangs forward

Shoulders slump forward

Constricted chest

Abdominal muscles are tense

SELF-HELP · EXERCISING

This person greatly benefits from sustained exercise. Running, dancing, and swimming deepen breathing and increase circulation while helping to build muscle tone and stamina. A roots and wings exercise (see page 39) will improve posture, and create a sense of stability and "backbone".

RELAXATION PROGRAM

PAGES 50-55

A SPECIALLY-DESIGNED program featuring massage suggestions, a postural alignment sequence, and a back massage helps the *victim type* find stability, release tension, and realign the body.

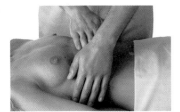

Chest Constriction in the collapsed, hollow chest area can be released by massaging the torso. This helps deepen the breathing and also boosts energy.

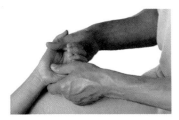

Arms Invigorating massage strokes increase vitality and strength in the arms and hands.

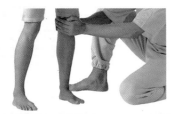

Knees Loosening stiff knees leads to a more balanced posture.

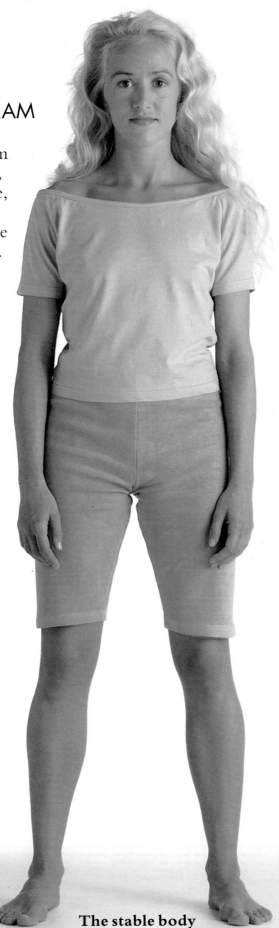

The stable body

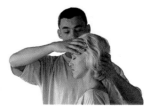

Neck Exercises to align the body lengthen the neck and release tension between head and neck.

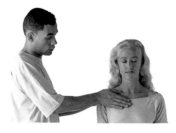

Shoulders A chest and shoulder stroke creates expansion and width. It also relieves a collapsed, contracted chest.

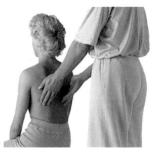

Back Deep back strokes loosen and extend the spine so that the head balances easily above it.

FURTHER RELAXATION

■ Relax the feet and legs. See *feet and ankles*; *legs and knees* pages 98-101.
■ Ease an over-stretched back. See *spine and lower back* pages 108-109.

THE WARRIOR
A · RIGID · BODY · AND · HOW · TO · RELAX · IT

Someone with the *warrior type* body almost certainly sets high standards for himself, and is ambitious, active, and assertive. Deep-rooted attitudes, including the need to win approval, and to display characteristics such as pride and strength, build up tension in the muscles, and this results in a posture that becomes rigid. This person's response to stress is one of fight or challenge, and the tight control exercised over the body, mind, and emotions inhibits spontaneity and prevents vulnerable feelings from being expressed.

CHARACTERISTICS

This type displays the classic "military" posture - head up, shoulders drawn back, chest inflated, rigid ramrod spine, a locked-back pelvis, and tight stiff legs. This creates specific points of tension and pain in the body. The *warrior type* can find it difficult to show vulnerability, weaknesses, and needs, and may hide love and hurt behind the tense, inflexible body.

SIGNS OF STRESS

■ The skin color can often look reddish, and both the feeling and tone of this body type indicate an overcharge of energy.
■ Tendency to inhale and hold the breath, rather than exhale with an easy letting go.
■ The chest is puffed-out and over-inflated.
■ The front of the body may be extended in an exaggerated way.
■ Muscles in the back are tight and shortened.
■ Tension in the lower back can inhibit this person's sexual spontaneity and cause feelings of frustration.

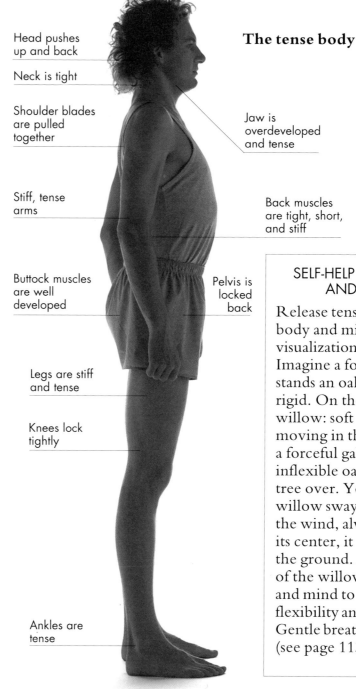

The tense body

Head pushes up and back

Neck is tight

Shoulder blades are pulled together

Stiff, tense arms

Buttock muscles are well developed

Legs are stiff and tense

Knees lock tightly

Ankles are tense

Jaw is overdeveloped and tense

Back muscles are tight, short, and stiff

Pelvis is locked back

SELF-HELP - THE WILLOW AND THE OAK

Release tension from both body and mind with this visualization exercise. Imagine a forest. On one side stands an oak tree: solid and rigid. On the other side is the willow: soft and yielding, moving in the breeze. When a forceful gale hits the inflexible oak, it blows the tree over. Yet because the willow sways and bends with the wind, always returning to its center, it remains rooted in the ground. Absorb the image of the willow into your body and mind to encourage flexibility and spontaneity. Gentle breathing exercises (see page 113) will also help.

RELAXATION PROGRAM

PAGES 58-65

A SEQUENCE OF LIFTING and releasing movements, and a beneficial chest and arm massage, will help the *warrior type* to relax more effectively, breathe more deeply, and become more trusting.

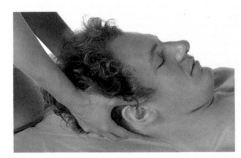

Head A head and neck lift is deeply relaxing for the *warrior type*. The head is supported and lifted up to create a stretch through the back of the neck.

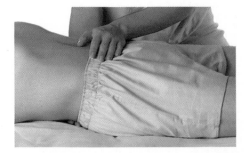

Pelvis A lower back and pelvis hold will create support and relaxation in this area.

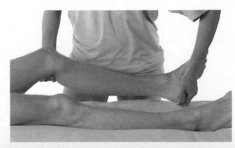

Legs Lifting and lowering the leg will also relax and release the hip.

The relaxed body

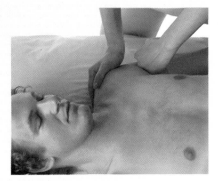

Upper arms An upper arm release using a deeper tissue massage stroke relaxes tension stored in the shoulder and tight upper arm muscles.

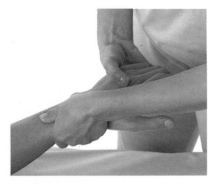

Lower arms Releasing tension in the forearm will ease tightness in the muscles and tissue that run between the elbow and wrist.

FURTHER RELAXATION

■ Massage the shoulders and neck. See *the guard* pages 47–49; *shoulders and neck* pages 103–105.
■ Ease the face (jaw and forehead). See *executive stress* pages 86–87; *head and face* pages 106–107.
■ Massage the lower back. See *spine and lower back* pages 108–109.
■ Relax the lower body. See *feet and ankles*; *legs and knees* pages 98–101.

THE INTELLECTUAL
A · DISORIENTATED · BODY · AND · HOW · TO · RELAX · IT

Frequently artistic, academic, or psychic, this person is often not at ease in the body and feels more comfortable when escaping into fantasy, imagination, or intellect. As a result, the *intellectual type* person may become out of touch with basic emotions and feelings, and can be physically uncoordinated. At the root of such an attitude is often a deep sense of insecurity, which causes the body's natural energy to contract inward to the core. This type of personality will create self-esteem by developing the imagination or intellectual abilities, and, living so much in the mind, may feel like a stranger in the body.

CHARACTERISTICS

Physically, there may be marked differences between the upper and lower body, the left and right sides, or the front and back, and energy is concentrated in the head. Emotionally, this person may find difficulty in developing close, intimate contact with others.

SIGNS OF STRESS

■ The skin is often pale and cold to the touch, muscle tone is tight and tense, and joint areas are contracted: all signs that energy has shrunk inward.
■ Upper and lower parts of the body are disconnected.
■ The posture of this body type is not aligned.
■ Body temperature may vary at the joint areas.
■ The head may seem to lead the whole body, and there is a tendency to walk and move as if lifting slightly off the ground.

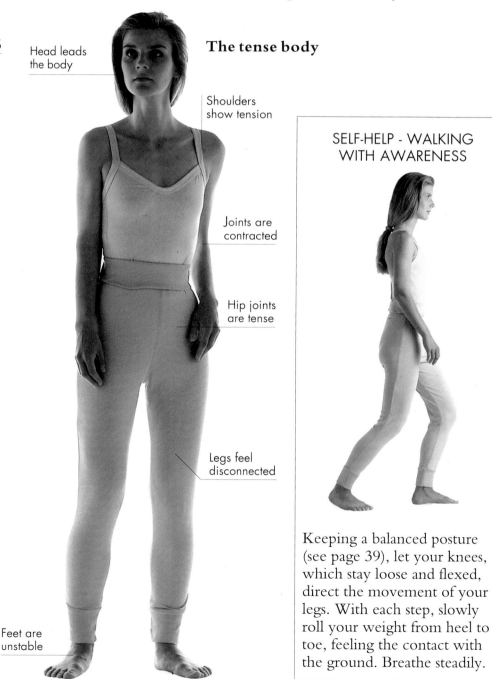

The tense body

Head leads the body

Shoulders show tension

Joints are contracted

Hip joints are tense

Legs feel disconnected

Feet are unstable

SELF-HELP - WALKING WITH AWARENESS

Keeping a balanced posture (see page 39), let your knees, which stay loose and flexed, direct the movement of your legs. With each step, slowly roll your weight from heel to toe, feeling the contact with the ground. Breathe steadily.

RELAXATION PROGRAM

PAGES 66-69

TO HELP THE BODY RELAX both emotionally and physically, each part in relationship with the other, a full body massage and balancing connection holds are very useful.

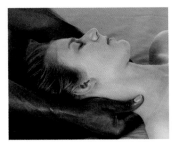

Neck Contracted areas of muscle release under massage strokes.

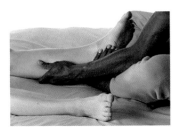

Legs and feet Strokes on the legs and feet bring a sense of grounding and balance to the whole body.

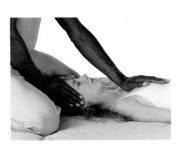

Head and heart A head-heart connection hold encourages calming feelings of integration.

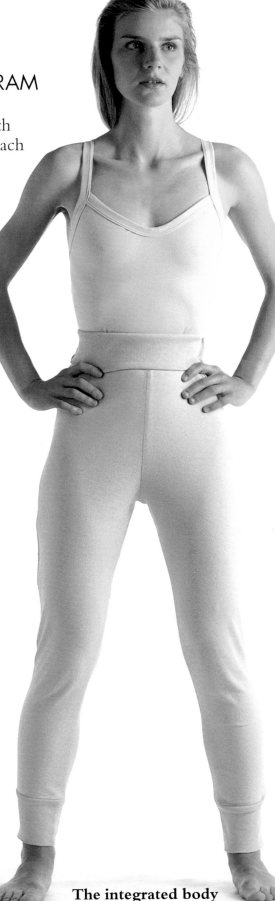

The integrated body

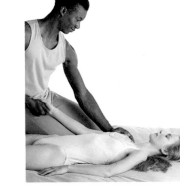

Shoulders and arms A shoulder–hand hold will relax the shoulder joint, and increase the flow of energy through the arm.

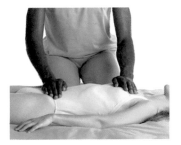

Heart and abdomen This hold connects the abdomen with the heart, which is the emotional center of the body.

FURTHER RELAXATION

■ All postural alignment work is beneficial before a massage or connection holds. See *roots and wings* pages 38–41.

■ Lifting and releasing movements ease tense joints and help realign posture. See *the warrior* pages 58–62.

THE SUPERMAN

A · MACHO · POSTURE · AND · HOW · TO · RELAX · IT

To be successful and happy it is important to have confidence in yourself and a strong sense of self-esteem. By understanding yourself and nurturing your potential, while accepting your vulnerabilities, you can develop these qualities. The "superman" or "superwoman", however, develops an image of strength both in body and personality based more on a fear of failure and the need to control others. In wanting to be the center of attention, and to dominate every situation, either by aggression, charm, or seduction, a physique is created (with its inevitable tension points) that enables this person to stay in control.

CHARACTERISTICS

The posture is often that of the classic macho man: top heavy, carrying strength in the chest and shoulders, but often narrow and contracted in the pelvis and stomach. Breathing is focused in the chest, and the reluctance to exhale is symptomatic of a fear of losing control and becoming vulnerable. Vital energy is drawn up the body to maintain strength and avoid vulnerable sexual feelings, which results in an overcharge of energy in the neck, head, and face.

SIGNS OF STRESS

■ The lower half of the body is out of proportion to the puffed-up upper half.
■ The legs of this body type can look surprisingly thin or weak.
■ The muscles of the diaphragm are constricted.

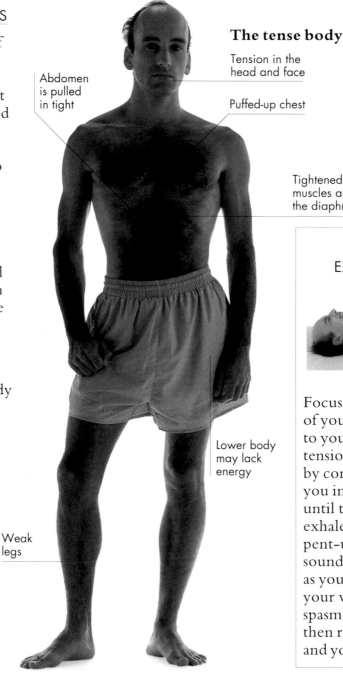

The tense body

Tension in the head and face

Abdomen is pulled in tight

Puffed-up chest

Tightened muscles around the diaphragm

Lower body may lack energy

Weak legs

SELF-HELP - EXPELLING TENSION

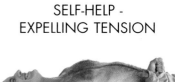

Focus attention on each part of your body, from your toes to your face. Exaggerate the tension in one area at a time by contracting the muscles as you inhale. Hold your breath until the body is forced to exhale and discharge the pent-up energy. Make a sound to express the release as you exhale. Now tighten your whole body as if in a spasm, hold the tension, and then release. Feel your body and your breathing relax.

RELAXATION PROGRAM
PAGES 72-77

LOOSENING TIGHT muscles in the abdominal region allows breathing to deepen, encouraging a connection with deeper emotions.

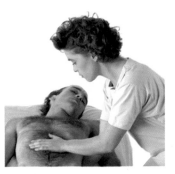

Solar plexus Helping the breathing to deepen, a connection hold is soothing and has an integrating effect.

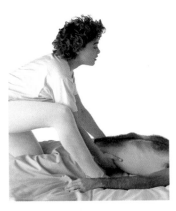

Lower back Tension in the muscles of the abdomen, and stress in the lower back, can be loosened by rocking.

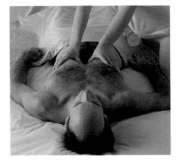

Rib cage Stretching and easing the muscle beneath the rib cage enhances the flow of breath in the body.

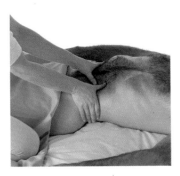

Abdomen The muscles in this area can be eased still further with a deep thumb rolling stroke.

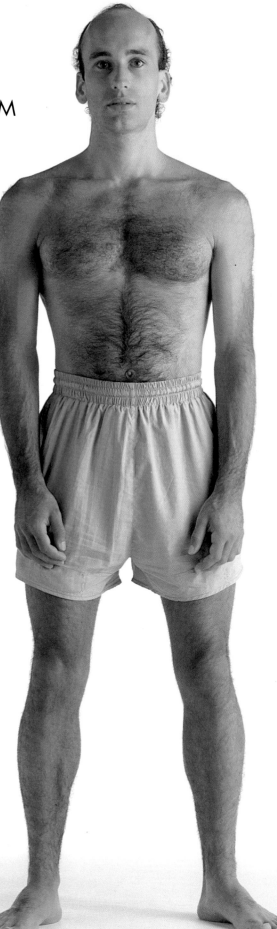

The relaxed body

FURTHER RELAXATION

■ Relax the lower body to allow tension to release downward. See *feet and ankles*; *legs and knees*; *pelvis and groin* pages 98-102.
■ Then massage the over-charged upper half of the body. See *shoulders and neck*; *head and face* pages 103-107.

THE STOIC

A · BURDENED · BODY · AND · HOW · TO · RELAX · IT

Freedom and choice are essential ingredients for health and happiness, and are reflected in a relaxed and vital mind and body. Occasionally in life, though, we feel dragged down by a lack of free choice. Feeling trapped in a boring job or an unfulfilling relationship, being overwhelmed by family responsibilities, going through financial hardship – all add to an inner sense of defeat, low self-esteem, and the feeling of being burdened by life. The sense of having a yoke around the neck, whether a passing phase or a deep-seated attitude developed early in life, creates a *stoic type* personality, which is marked by feelings of self-sacrifice, endurance, and frustration. The resulting stress patterns create a physique bowed down with tension.

CHARACTERISTICS

Over time, a burdened attitude creates physical tensions in the body as natural vitality is pushed downward. This body type feels heavy, and the stoicism may be accompanied by sighing and complaining. Frustration, stubbornness, and rage can become trapped in the leg muscles.

SIGNS OF STRESS

- Muscle tone tends to be flaccid, and the skin cold to the touch.
- Weight and tension build up in the jaw, neck and upper back muscles.
- Shoulders stoop as this person metaphorically carries the weight of the world on her shoulders.
- Chronic tension shortens the torso and pushes it downward.
- Pelvis slumps forward, adding strain to the lower half of the body.

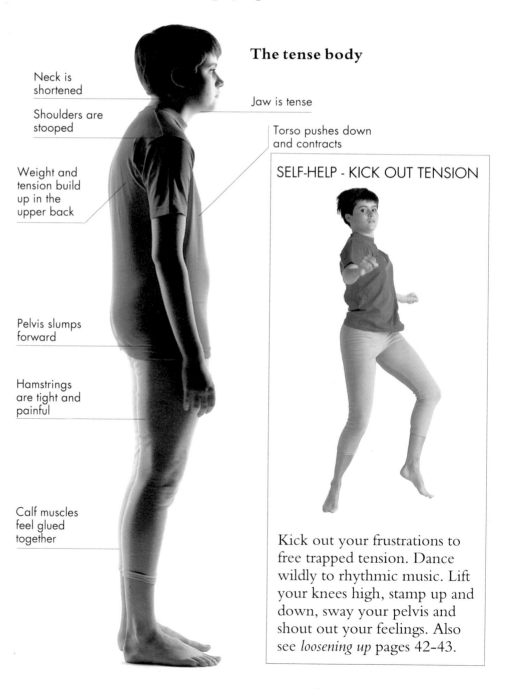

The tense body

Neck is shortened

Shoulders are stooped

Weight and tension build up in the upper back

Jaw is tense

Torso pushes down and contracts

Pelvis slumps forward

Hamstrings are tight and painful

Calf muscles feel glued together

SELF-HELP - KICK OUT TENSION

Kick out your frustrations to free trapped tension. Dance wildly to rhythmic music. Lift your knees high, stamp up and down, sway your pelvis and shout out your feelings. Also see *loosening up* pages 42-43.

RELAXATION PROGRAM
PAGES 78-83

A SEQUENCE OF MASSAGE, deep bodywork, and movement will help the *stoic type* regain vitality and self-expression, and release tension.

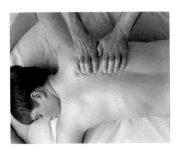

Top of spine The long muscles of the back can be loosened up with a palpitation stroke.

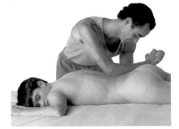

Back Tightness in the muscles surrounding the vertebrae is released by using a longer, deeper stretch stroke.

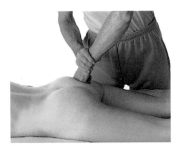

Buttocks and lower back The heel of the hand or flat of the knuckles is used to alleviate deep-rooted tension.

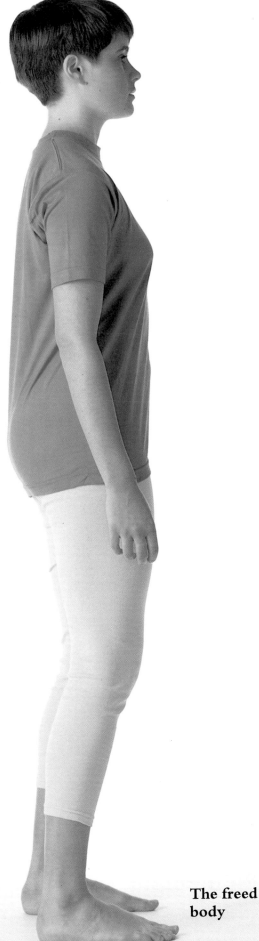

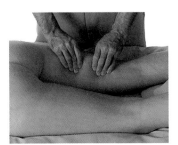

Thighs Squeezing, rocking, and lifting the muscle away from the bone relieve heaviness.

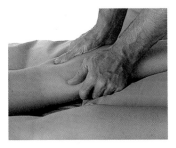

Calves Stretch strokes using pressure from the heels of the hands ease glued-together muscles.

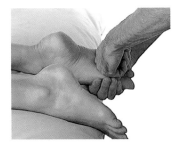

Feet Knuckle stretch strokes loosen tension and increase flexibility.

The freed body

FURTHER RELAXATION
- Ease the neck. See *shoulders and neck* pages 103-105.
- Massage the chest. See *the guard* page 46.
- Relax the stomach. See *the superman* pages 72-75.

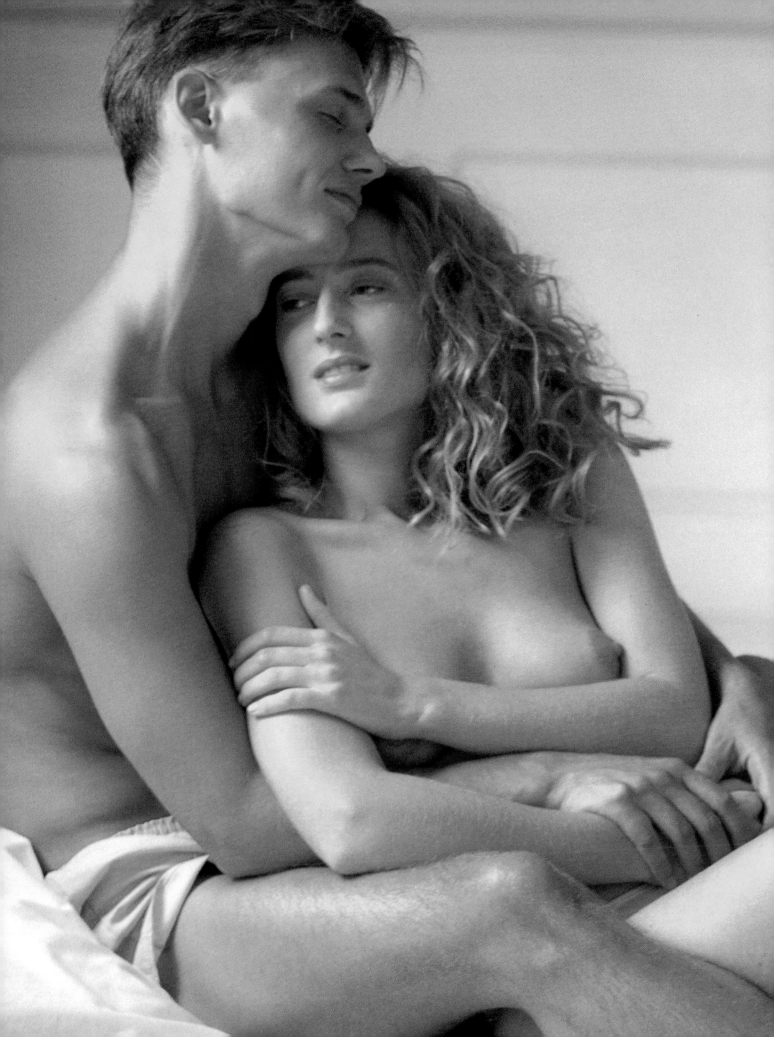

2
RELAXATION TACTICS

The art of relaxing and of balancing activity
and rest has become an essential skill in
our modern, fast-paced world. This section
suggests beneficial ways to restore vitality
and equilibrium to body and mind,
using the techniques of massage,
breath awareness, body alignment
and loosening up.

MASSAGE
AND · THE · IMPORTANCE · OF · TOUCH

Massage is a science and an art. The beauty of the skill is that your touch and strokes bring gentle, beneficial changes to your massage partner, while they nourish you and allow you to explore your own creativity. The caring touch of your hands relaxes and soothes away stress and tension from body and mind. It also stimulates and invigorates the physiological system, and restores energy

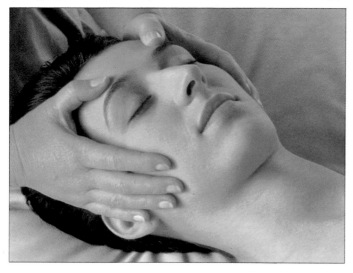

Bringing your full attention and care to the quality of your touch does much to relax and nourish your partner.

and vitality. Massage is just as rewarding for the person who gives it. By learning where and how to touch the body, by becoming sensitive and caring, and by gaining an understanding of the causes of tension and the ways to release it, you will become more aware of your own body, your breathing and your emotional patterns. This in turn allows you to find greater relaxation and harmony within yourself. To give a good massage you need to discover the balance between developing your technique and trusting your intuitive responses to your partner's needs. The suggestions below will help you prepare for and give a sensitive, satisfying massage.

PREPARATION FOR MASSAGE

Always give a massage in a warm, welcoming room. Keep the lighting soft and diffused, and make sure the room temperature remains at about 70 °C. Remove any clutter from the area in which you are working, as this might distract you and your partner, and impede your movement around your partner's body. Take off any jewelry that might catch on the skin, and ask your partner to do the same. It is important to have privacy throughout the massage session.

MASSAGE ACCESSORIES

Before starting to massage, make sure that everything you need for the session is ready and within easy reach. You will need either oil or lotion in a bottle that will not tip or spill easily (see page 34). Place a warm, clean sheet on the massage table or mattress for your partner to lie on, and keep another sheet ready to cover her with while she rests and assimilates the massage at the end of the session. Use large, clean towels to cover any parts of the body that you are not massaging immediately. Body temperature quickly drops when lying still, and it is important to keep your partner warm and relaxed. Some people are happy to be completely exposed during a massage; others feel more secure if they are partially covered: learn to assess your partner's needs. Towels can also be used to wipe excess oil from the body at the end of the massage.

Pillows placed under the body ease tension and loosen tight muscles as well as making your partner more comfortable while lying down. Put a pillow under his knees when your partner is on his back; just below the knees when on his stomach. A thin pillow placed beneath the abdomen eases a sway back; and when placed below the chest, it helps someone with a tense upper body. Consider investing in a massage table if you intend to massage regularly. It enables you to stand correctly and comfortably while working, preventing back pain and strains, and allows you to change position easily.

Massage tables can be built to measure. Find the correct height for you by standing by the table, your arms hanging by your sides. Your knuckles should just skim the surface of the padding. Buy a sturdy table, especially if you intend to use a lot of movement in a massage or wish to climb onto the table to apply deeper pressure. A massage table can be built to stand for use, and to fold for easy moving and storage. Alternatively, you can massage on a padded base on the floor. A piece of foam or a thin mattress, blankets or sleeping bags, all covered with a clean sheet, will suffice. Make sure you also kneel on a padded surface. If you massage on the floor, take even more care of your posture so that you do not strain your back. Read the hints below on keeping your body comfortable before starting to massage from this position.

HOW TO USE YOUR BODY

In massage it is of paramount importance that while you are taking care of someone else's body, you also look after your own. If you feel uncomfortable giving a massage, pain, discomfort, strain and tiredness follow, and these will adversely affect the quality of your strokes. Use the roots and wings body awareness exercise on page 39 and let it remind you constantly to keep your back straight, shoulders wide, and your neck and head balanced and in line with your spine.

When standing at a table, place your feet apart and firmly on the ground, with your knees relaxed. Tip forward from your hips, bend in the knees, and let your leg muscles support all your weight. When kneeling on the floor to massage, keep your knees apart to give yourself support and balance, or keep one knee bent with your foot on the floor to provide leverage and to make movement easier. Do not hunch over your strokes or twist yourself into an uncomfortable position. Face in the direction of your stroke as much as possible, do not overstretch, and never attempt a movement or a lift, or try a stroke, that puts your body at risk of strain. To add pressure to a stroke, lean into it with your whole body weight.

Always breathe deeply and fully while you massage. Staying conscious of your own breathing gives you energy and vitality, and ensures your massage stays alive, refreshing, and yet relaxing. This flow of energy will transmit to your partner, enhancing trust and relaxation. If you feel tense or tired during a massage, stop for a while. Place your hands gently on your partner in a calm connecting hold (see page 67) while you breathe deeply and relax your body and mind.

Prepare yourself emotionally and physically before giving a massage. Separate yourself from the day's events by being quietly meditative, even if only for a few minutes. Consciously relax your entire body. Then bring your whole attention into the session as if it were a meditation. In this way both you and your partner will gain tremendous benefit from the experience. In a good massage giver and receiver will feel equally nourished, relaxed, and revitalized.

OILS AND LOTIONS

Using a suitable oil or lotion enables your hands to glide over the skin and mould to the body's contours. Massage lotion, easily absorbed by the skin, is particularly good to use with stronger, deeper strokes. Light nut and vegetable oils, such as grapeseed, olive, sunflower, apricot kernel and soya, are good carrier oils. Mix richer, more expensive oils, such as avocado and sweet almond, into them, or try a few drops of an essential oil, extracted from herbs and plants. Used in aromatherapy, essential oils have beneficial effects on the body, mind and emotions. Keep oils in plastic bottles with a narrow top and stopper, store in a cool place and renew frequently. Before smoothing oil onto the body, rub a few drops between your palms to warm it. Use only enough oil for your hands to slide smoothly. Too much feels sticky and uncomfortable on the skin, and you will be unable to clasp the flesh fully or add pressure to deeper or more invigorating strokes.

THE RHYTHM AND SEQUENCE OF STROKES

Smooth, flowing strokes are the best way to apply oil or lotion to your partner's skin when starting a massage. Make sure that the entire surface of the area you are massaging is covered with oil or lotion.

Once you have learned the different massage strokes, it is important to understand how to apply them to create a flowing and satisfying massage. The *glossary of strokes* (see pages 119–125) gives basic ideas on how to relax, invigorate, and stimulate the body by using your hands and strokes in different ways. There are no rules for giving a massage. You can begin on whichever part of the body feels right to you and your partner, but most people find it easier to start on the back, the least threatening area of the body. Starting a

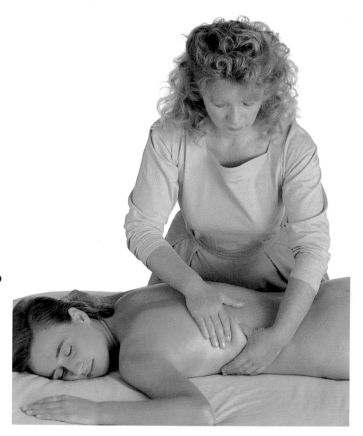

By learning how, where and when to apply different strokes you can create many effects.

massage here gives your partner time to trust your hands and relax. Releasing tension from the back benefits the whole body and makes it easier to massage more vulnerable areas. Establishing a rhythm and flow in massage prevents you from jumping between areas of the body, or strokes, in a disjointed way. To enhance wholeness, connect one part of the body to another. Begin with relaxing strokes, then work deeper to release tension. Finally, use soft strokes to harmonize the different effects. Practice makes perfect in massage, and soon your hands will respond intuitively to the needs of your partner's body. First learn the techniques, develop the sensitivity, and then trust your feelings.

DEEPENING YOUR STROKES

Deeper tissue strokes release emotional and muscular tension. As well as hands, thumbs and fingers, the forearm, knuckles, heel of the hand, or flat of the elbow penetrate the tissue gently. Try them when familiar with your partner's body, and when confident with softer, more basic strokes.

USING DEEPER STROKES

■ Prepare the area with soft, rounded strokes.
■ Be sensitive to your partner's ability to relax under deepened pressure. Always check that the pressure is comfortable, and lighten it if your partner tenses.
■ Deeper strokes should not be rushed. Move very slowly, working with your partner's breathing and the willingness of the muscles to let you penetrate.
■ Do not start or finish a deep stroke abruptly. Add pressure gradually, and lessen it as you complete the movement for a smooth finish.
■ When using knuckles or elbows in a stretch, use the flat surface. Do not penetrate muscles with sharp, bony parts of your body.
■ Tension forms to protect the body and will release when ready. Always respect a person's tension and never demand or expect change.

SPEAKING TO YOUR PARTNER

Massage and touch are a language. Your hands interpret messages from your partner's body, and transmit care and relaxation. Silence deepens this experience. Yet at times it feels right to urge your partner to become more aware of the potential for even greater relaxation. Introducing verbal suggestions at an appropriate time, in conjunction with touch, movements and strokes, helps this process. In massage, words act as a subtle seduction to help the body relax naturally; never let them imply criticism of tension.

USING WORDS

■ Placing your hands on your partner and suggesting that she focuses her breathing on them expands the flow of breath into the area and restores balance and inner calm. See *the intellectual* pages 67-69.
■ Ask your partner to breathe into slower, deeper strokes, especially those that stretch and release tight bands of muscle (see *the stoic* pages 80-81). This helps her to let tension dissolve consciously.
■ Verbal directions help your partner visualize beneficial changes (see *roots and wings* pages 40-41; *the victim* pages 50-53). The images will remind your partner of a relaxed posture when tension returns.
■ Urge your partner to let you take the weight of his body and move it without his help (see *the warrior* pages 58-62). This helps relax control. Use simple phrases, e.g. "let me take the weight of your head".

WHEN NOT TO MASSAGE

Massage is almost always beneficial, but there are times when it is advisable not to massage.
■ Never use massage to treat a medical or psychiatric condition without taking the advice of a qualified medical practitioner.
■ Consult a doctor if you have doubts about the suitability of massage for any person or condition.
■ Do not massage someone with a high fever, or an infected or contagious skin condition.

■ Never massage septic swellings, such as boils, or any undiagnosed inflammation or lumps.
■ Do not massage over recent scar tissue, fresh wounds, or varicose veins.
■ If your partner has acute back pain, or any unexplained painful areas, advise him to see a doctor before receiving a massage.
■ If your partner has thrombosis, phlebitis, or heart problems, never massage without a doctor's consent.

BREATHING
TO · RELAX · BODY · MIND · AND · SOUL

Breath is the food of life. Breathe correctly and you nourish your body, mind and soul. When unimpeded by tension or control, breath flows through the body like a wave, cleansing and purifying each part of you. As you inhale it brings vital oxygen into your blood, feeding each cell and tissue. As you exhale it expels the toxic wastes from your body. Breath helps you pulsate with vitality and energy, so that your body stays relaxed, your mind continues to be open and alert, and your emotions remain in equilibrium. Using breath in conjunction with touch enhances the healing quality of massage as it creates beneficial changes not only in the body, but also in the mind and emotions.

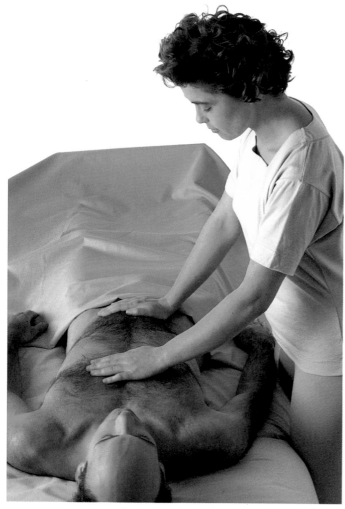

BREATHING FOR RELAXATION

While breathing is an automatic function of the body, learning how to breathe correctly and consciously will help you in many ways. In times of stress and anxiety, slow and deliberate breathing which reaches deep down into your abdomen will soothe and calm you; while deep, full breathing will replenish your energy and vitality when you feel tired and fatigued. Breathing into an area of the body that is tense or painful will relax it and ease the discomfort; and in times of emotional distress, conscious breathing will help you to discharge your pent-up feelings in a very natural way.

BREATHING AND MEDITATION

Many schools of meditation have used breath awareness as a way to gain peace of mind and relax the body. Some of these practices are based on ancient Eastern traditions, but their benefits are increasingly recognized and used to combat the stresses of modern life in the Western world. When practiced daily for even short periods, meditation enables you to find a sense of stillness and inner calm.

BREATHING EXERCISES

- Breathing correctly to enhance relaxation and to release tension. See page 113.
- Breathing techniques used in meditation. See page 112.

- Breathing and touch. See *the intellectual* pages 67–69, and *ways to calm* page 113.

To deepen relaxation, place your hands on your friend's body and urge him to breathe fully. ◁

Sit quietly and witness the movement of breath as you inhale and exhale during meditation. ▷

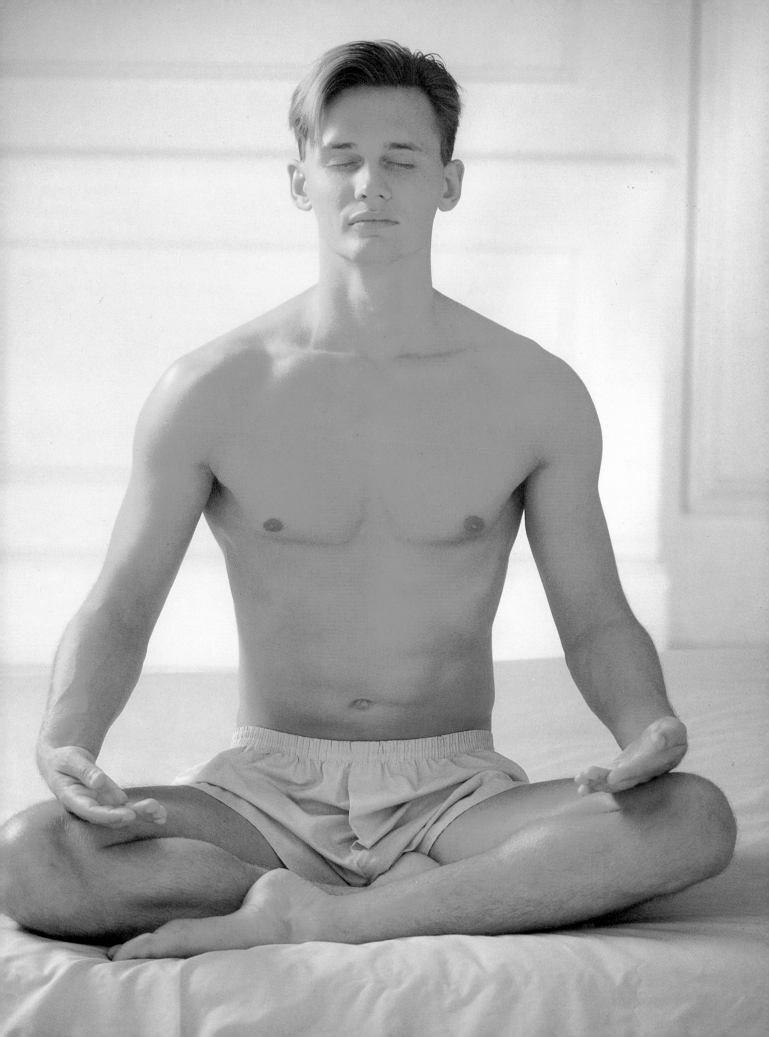

ROOTS & WINGS
EXERCISES · TO · BALANCE · THE · BODY

The body is the best place to begin when freeing yourself from habits that restrict you physically and emotionally. Learn how to bring your body in line and develop a relaxed posture, instead of tensing or collapsing under the force of gravity. By doing so you can release the muscular armor that surrounds withheld emotions and restricts you from living life to the full. The following visualization and awareness techniques, together with massage strokes, help develop the concept of "roots" and "wings" in your body, so that you can find balance and harmony within yourself, grace in your movements, and freedom from tension and pain. In this way, you become more flexible and spontaneous. You are able to respond to stress, to discharge tension naturally, and then relax.

ROOTS

Think of a tree, its roots growing down into the earth, spreading deep and wide to provide support. Developing an awareness of your own roots will provide your body with a firm, solid foundation. In physical terms, when you allow the lower half of your body to send its weight down toward the ground, your upper body is given the balance and support it needs. Emotionally, allowing your roots to develop will enable you to feel more secure with your feelings. It also allows you to stay in touch with your real needs, and helps you stand your ground when faced with stress and challenges.

WINGS

Once you feel grounded in your lower body — the pelvis, buttocks, legs, and feet — you will have the support needed to extend yourself upward and to align your spine, neck, and head like correctly balanced building blocks. By lengthening the spine and neck, widening and releasing through the chest and shoulders, and carrying the heavy weight of the head correctly, you will avoid rigidity or collapse in the posture, and encourage your body and spirit to move with fluidity and freedom. When finding your roots and wings, you may experience warm, tingling sensations as your cramped muscles and contracted joints release their tension. Feelings may also arise as various parts of the body let go of their protective physical armor.

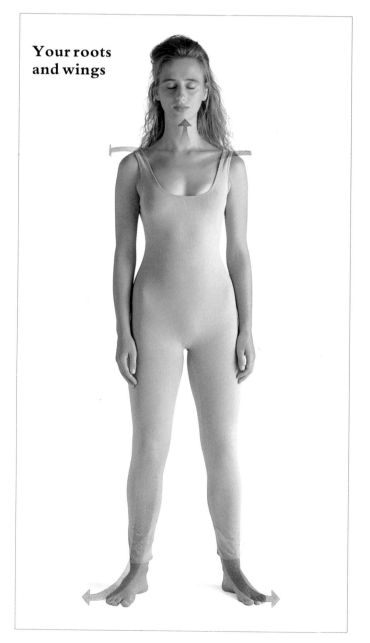

Your roots and wings

FINDING YOUR ROOTS AND WINGS

SHARE THIS EXERCISE with your massage partner, especially after a massage, taking turns to guide each other through the wonderful release it allows the standing body. Or use it at any time when you wish to realign and bring balance to the body, and release emotional and physical tension.

1 Close your eyes and focus on your own breathing. Place the feet parallel, facing ahead and at shoulder-width or a comfortable distance apart. Feel the stability of your feet on the ground, spread out your toes and distribute your weight evenly over the feet.

2 Unlock your knees and notice how the pelvis immediately gives you more support.

3 Drop the weight of your buttocks down through the leg muscles. Imagine that you have a heavy tail attached to the base of your spine. Let this heavy tail sink down toward the floor.

4 Breathe down deep into the pelvis, buttocks and genitals, then down through the thighs, legs and feet into the ground. Imagine that you are growing deep, wide roots.

5 Imagine energy is flowing up through your torso, and your spine is lengthening. Let it create space between each of your vertebrae.

6 Allow your neck to lengthen and to release upward from the shoulders, aligning with the spine. Let the head float up like a balloon, the spine as its string. Your head should float as if on a cushion of air.

7 Feel stability in the lower body; grace, lightness and mobility in your upper body.

8 Focus on a central point in the chest. Feel your shoulders and chest widen out from this point, like wings. Let the arms lengthen from your shoulders, and your hands relax.

9 Stand easy, breathing softly and deeply. Imagine your roots and wings as you move.

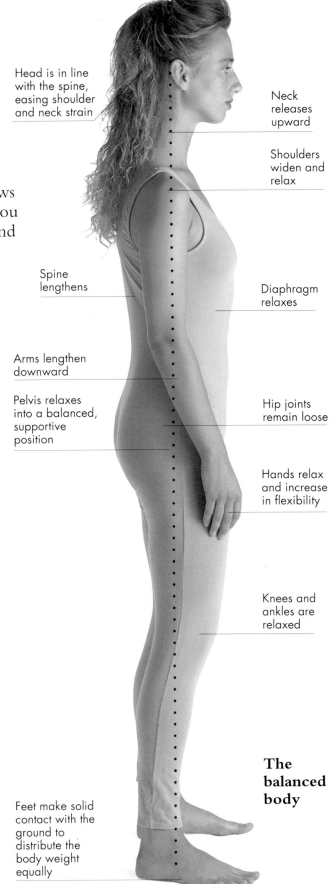

Head is in line with the spine, easing shoulder and neck strain

Neck releases upward

Shoulders widen and relax

Spine lengthens

Diaphragm relaxes

Arms lengthen downward

Pelvis relaxes into a balanced, supportive position

Hip joints remain loose

Hands relax and increase in flexibility

Knees and ankles are relaxed

Feet make solid contact with the ground to distribute the body weight equally

The balanced body

A ROOTS AND WINGS MASSAGE

UNTIL YOU ENCOURAGE your partner to relax and lie comfortably, some areas of the body may be too cramped to benefit from massage. The strokes below will help your partner to release physical tension and feel much more open and relaxed. Use them as a session in themselves, at the start of a massage, or at any time during a massage to release any postural tension. While doing these strokes, use the phrases suggested below to describe the direction of the movement and the release of the body. This makes your partner more aware of changes in her body during and even after the session. Use the verbal directions as gentle suggestions, not to control or criticize your partner, and let them remind you to keep your own posture relaxed as well. Work on one side of the front of the body, then the other. End the session by holding the feet for a while to balance and connect both sides of the body.

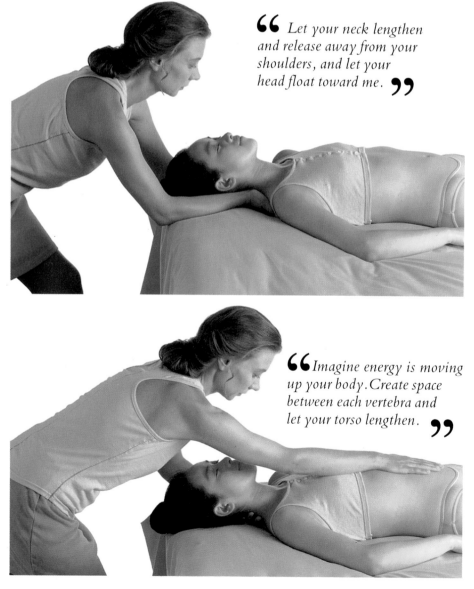

66 *Let your neck lengthen and release away from your shoulders, and let your head float toward me.* 99

66*Imagine energy is moving up your body. Create space between each vertebra and let your torso lengthen.* 99

HEAD AND NECK

Stand behind your friend's head. Slide your hands under the back and between the shoulder blades, fingers pointing down each side of the spine. Let the base of the neck rest on your palms and your heels. When your friend relaxes, draw your hands slowly up the neck. Lift the head slightly at the hairline and draw out of the hair. Rest the head on the base of the skull, using a thin book or pillow if the neck is still contracted. ◁

SHOULDERS

Place both your hands over the shoulders, fingers pointing to the chest. Gently push the shoulders back to the mattress and release them slowly after your friend has inhaled and exhaled three times.

TORSO AND SPINE

Place your right hand as far down the body as you can. Do not over-stretch. As the abdomen relaxes, glide your hand slowly up to the top of the breastbone. Release the head and neck again, as above. ◁

> *Let your shoulder release away from your chest. Now allow the arm to lengthen away from the shoulder as I pull down. Relax your elbow and wrist, hands and fingers.*

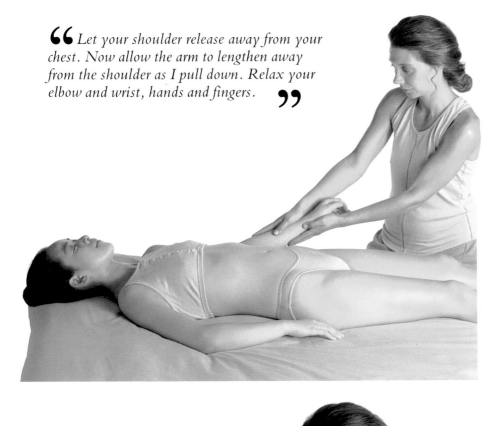

> *Allow your lower back to melt into the mattress. Feel your pelvis and hip release and your leg lengthen. Let the feeling of length move down to your toes.*

Position yourself to make a forward and backward movement

CHEST, SHOULDERS AND ARMS

Face your friend's left side. Lift the shoulder and slide your right hand under the shoulder blade, fingers pointing toward the spine. Place your left hand on the upper chest, fingers pointing toward the breastbone. Wait for the shoulder to relax. When ready, draw both your hands out to the shoulder. Then flex your wrists and move your body to face your friend's shoulder. Stretch-pull down the arm and out of the fingers. ◁

RIB CAGE

Slide your right hand under the back, beneath the lower rib cage, fingers pointing toward the spine. Place your left hand parallel, on top of the rib cage. Encourage the area to drop down by slightly depressing the upper hand. Then slowly draw your hands out to the side of the body.

PELVIS AND LEGS

Face the left hip. Slide your right hand under the lower back, your left hand under the inner thigh, with fingers pointing toward the buttocks. When the area relaxes, draw your right hand down and behind the buttocks until even with your left hand. Then slide your right hand around to the top of the thigh. Stretch-pull down the leg using both hands. Pause at the knee, step back, and continue the stretch down the leg. Draw out of the foot. ◁

LOOSENING UP
MOVEMENT · AND · EXERCISE · FOR · VITALITY

Exercise and movement are important ingredients for health and happiness. Keeping your body flexible will help you to move easily and gracefully, release tension, and bring you the joy and liberation of both vitality and relaxation. Find the methods of exercise that suit you, then introduce them into your daily life. Swimming and walking exercise and revitalize the whole body gently but fully. Other aerobic activities such as running or cycling strengthen the muscles and boost the cardiovascular system. Stretch and yoga movements release tension and keep you supple and toned, while bringing a harmony between body and mind. And martial arts like t'ai chi or karate build up inner power and stability. To increase your flexibility and release tension from the major joints in your body, use the exercises below, keeping a relaxed and balanced stance throughout (see page 39).

RELEASING THE HEAD AND NECK

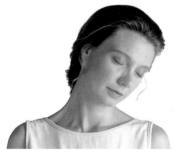

1 Focus on the hollow spot that lies at the top of your spine and below your skull. Use this spot as a pivot point, and imagine that your head is becoming free from the neck. Slowly drop your head forward, and then begin to roll it gently around to the left. ◁

2 Roll your head backward, then continue to the right.

3 Let the head fall to the front of the body. Repeat this circular motion five times, then reverse it to the right. Bring the head up in line with the spine.

FREEING THE SHOULDERS

1 Allow your arms and hands to hang loosely from your shoulders, keeping your elbows and wrists relaxed. Focus on your right shoulder and, as you inhale, start to lift your right arm up slowly.

2 Feel the stretching movement in your shoulder joint as you raise your right arm up high above your head. ◁

3 Breathe out gently while you slowly lower your right arm back down behind your right shoulder. ◁

4 Feeling the rotary movement of your shoulder joint, repeat the movement five times with the right arm and shoulder, then five times with the left. When your shoulders feel relaxed, make five full rotations with both arms at once.

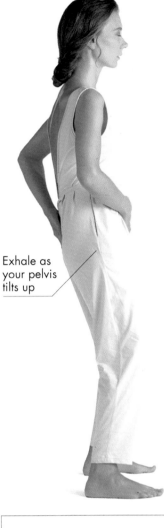

Exhale as your pelvis tilts up

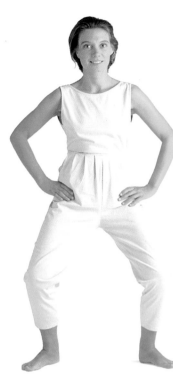

RELAXING THE PELVIS

1 Focus on and isolate these movements in your pelvis, all the time breathing deeply into your abdomen. Place your right hand over your lower abdomen, left hand on the base of your spine. Inhale and tilt your pelvis back.

2 Exhale while you slowly release your pelvis forward. Repeat this gentle movement ten times to build up a steady rocking motion in your pelvic area. ◁

3 Place your hands over your hips and then rotate your pelvis to make five full circles, first moving to the left, then to the right.

FLEXING THE KNEES

1 Stand with your legs apart, feet turned out at a comfortable angle, and hands on your hips. Bend at the knees, and drop your weight down through the body. Keep your knees in line with your feet, and make sure that your feet are placed firmly on the ground. ◁

2 Straighten up again and then repeat the movement five times.

ROTATING THE ANKLES

Use a chair or wall for balance if necessary. Bend your left knee to lift your left foot off the ground. Rotate the ankle five times to the left, then to the right. Repeat the rotations with the right ankle.

DANCING FOR FREEDOM

Dance acts as a massage for the body and mind, and it is one of the most enjoyable and effective ways to free all levels of tension. Use the dynamic movements to experience vitality, vibrancy and joy, which can be held in check by tight muscles and contracted joints. Dancing will stretch and tone the muscles, while it helps to invigorate the cardiovascular and nervous systems. It will also allow you to express yourself freely. Find a private place to dance, and do so with or without music in an abandoned way. Let your body move and sway, swing your head and loosen your arms and shoulders by letting them open wide and freely. As you dance, consciously free areas of tension within your body, and deepen your breathing. This will awaken your vitality. When you feel exhausted, lie down and relax, and sense how alive and vibrant your body feels. Hear your heart beating, feel your pulse throbbing, and the breath moving through your whole body.

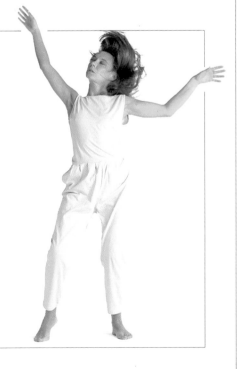

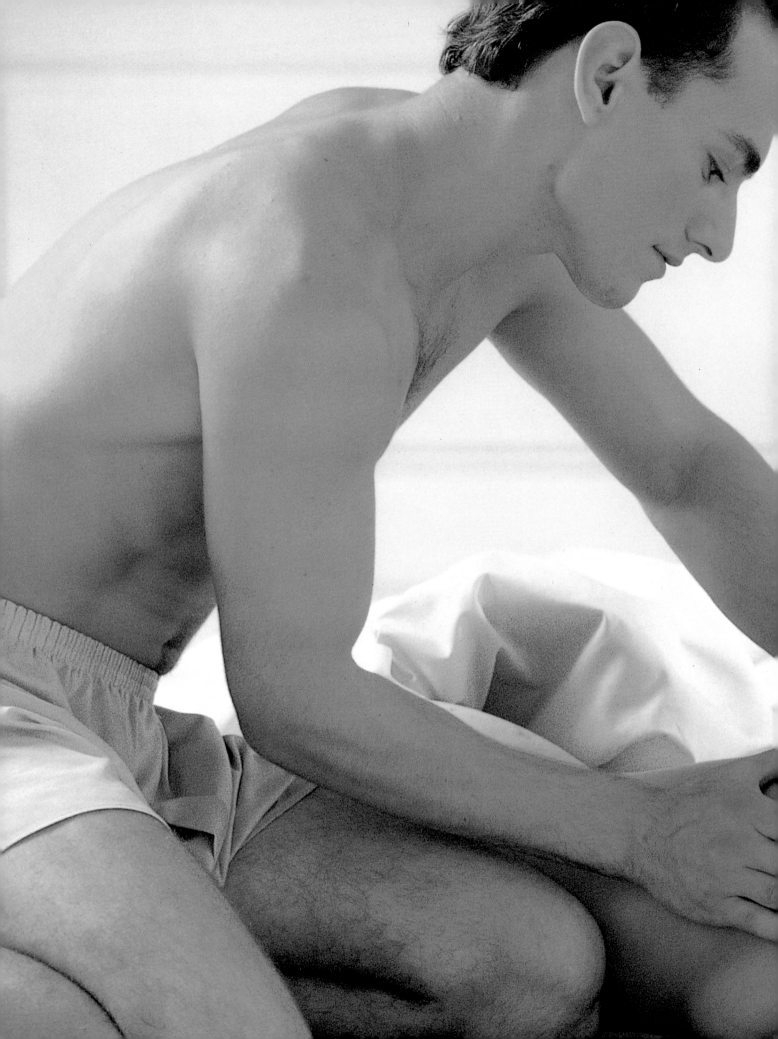

3
BODY TYPE PROGRAMS

Relaxing massage strokes and gentle touches can unlock the physical and psychological tensions rooted within us all. These specially devised massage sequences, using techniques specific to each body type, release tension by focusing on particular stress patterns.

THE GUARD
A · PROGRAM · FOR · RELAXATION

By gently manipulating the muscles you will see tension miraculously melt away from the *guard type*, who responds especially well to massage. As his defensive physical armor softens, and his body relaxes under your strokes, so his breathing deepens and natural vitality returns. Relieve pain in tight, sore spots by massaging the key tension areas of this body type: the neck, shoulders, chest, and back. The massage strokes below, for the chest and shoulders, bring relief and deep relaxation to these tense areas.

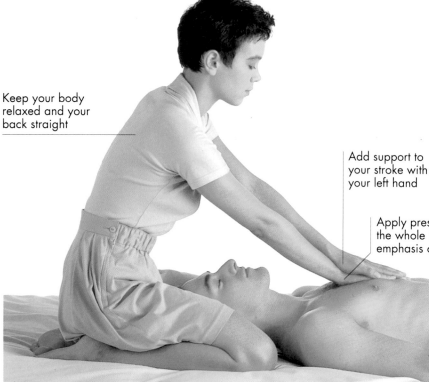

Keep your body relaxed and your back straight

Add support to your stroke with your left hand

Apply pressure from the whole hand with emphasis on the heel

RELEASING THE CHEST

1 Position yourself behind your partner's head. Place your right hand over the lower part of the breastbone and focus on his breathing. Rest your left hand over the right to add support to your stroke. Draw your hands up over the breastbone. ◁

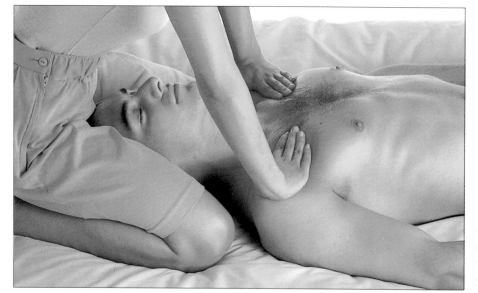

2 At the top of the breastbone separate the hands and slide toward the shoulders, thumb above, index finger below the collarbone. Sweep around the shoulders toward the back. Pull the heels into the back of the shoulder muscles. Swing fingers and palms along the spine. ◁

3 Sink your fingertips gently into the neck muscle as you draw the hands up. Lift the head a little at the hairline and pull out through the hair. For deeper relaxation, repeat the sequence.

46

SHOULDER ROCKING

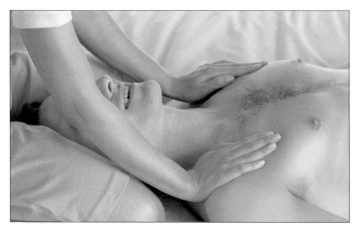

Remain in the same position. Place both hands over the shoulders, fingers pointing down the chest, heels on the shoulder ridge. Push the left shoulder down and out. Slowly release pressure as you repeat the movement on the other shoulder. Set up a rhythmic rocking in both shoulders.

RELAXING THE UPPER CHEST

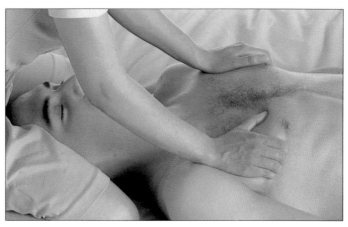

Position yourself behind your partner's head. To knead the tight upper chest muscles, anchor your fingertips lightly alongside the armpits. Then press from the heels, rhythmically sliding one hand at a time down from the collarbone to the armpit. Knead well to dissipate tension.

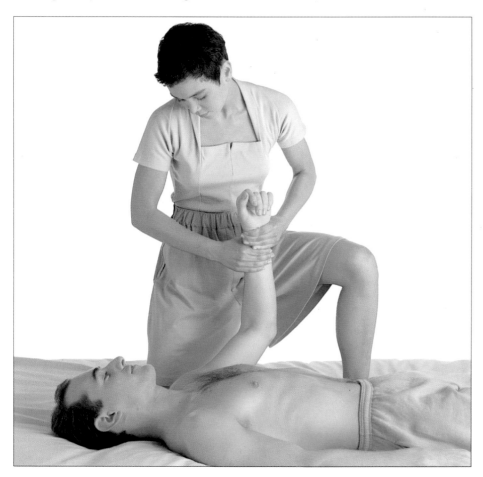

SHOULDER JOINT RELEASE

Move to your partner's side. Clasp the wrist securely with both your hands. Lift the arm and bring it away from the body, keeping the elbow flexed. Rock the arm to create a wave-like motion through the arm into the shoulder joint. Continue to move the arm around gently while rocking the shoulder joint, then lower it to the mattress. Remind your partner to let you do all the moving. Repeat the movement on the other arm.

BACK MASSAGE

Shoulders that habitually rise uncomfortably high into the neck, or round toward the chest, cause tension all through the back. This sequence of strokes, repeated on both sides of the body, counters back pain, dispelling tension from the shoulder blades and neck, as well as relaxing the tightened muscles that support the spine. Starting with your partner lying on his front, relax the back with basic strokes (see page 120), then slowly stretch the long muscles along the spine, before gently rocking away tension in the shoulder blades. Use soft, soothing touches between the deeper strokes.

SPINE AND SHOULDER STRETCH

Bend your knee to support your weight

Use the flat of your hand, with increased pressure in the heel

Move up alongside the spine

1 Position yourself by the lower back, and place your left hand on it. Add weight with your right hand and slowly slide up. △

2 Glide firmly across the shoulder muscles, taking the stroke a little way down and out through the arm.

3 Use your fingers and thumbs to massage tight areas around the shoulder blade and base of the neck (see page 123).

RELAXING THE SHOULDER BLADES

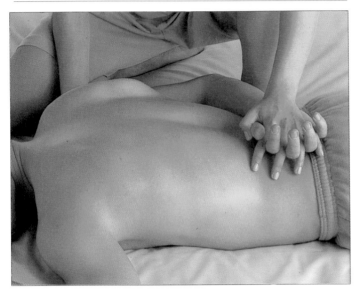

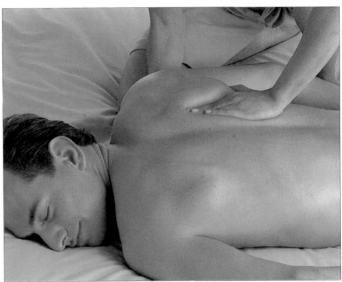

1 Make sure your fingernails are short if you try this sequence. Position yourself by your partner's right side. Create a lift in the shoulder blade by placing his forearm gently across his back, and supporting it with your left hand. Slip your right hand under the shoulder, and gently rock it up and down. Rest the arm back on the mattress.

2 Slip your right hand under the right shoulder and raise it to lift the blade slightly. Bring the left hand directly below the shoulder blade at the side of the rib cage. Glide your left hand around and slightly under the bone, stretching the tissue with your fingertips. Continue over the top of the shoulder and slightly down the arm. Repeat three times, penetrating deeper under the shoulder blade.

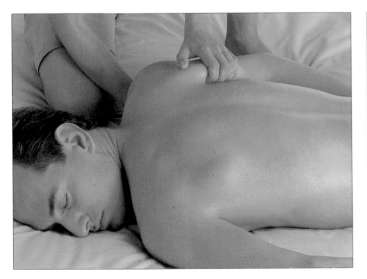

3 Grip the base of the raised shoulder blade just under the ridge with your fingertips, and rock gently and rhythmically back and forth. Repeat this movement further up the blade. Now use some soothing strokes to relax the shoulder area.

FINISHING TOUCHES

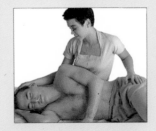

At the end of the session, enhance your partner's relaxation by asking him to rest on his side as you softly place your hands on his head and his hip. This hold will increase his sense of trust and security, enabling him to relax into his vulnerability.

THE VICTIM
A · PROGRAM · FOR · RELAXATION

A relaxing massage gently eases tension from overstrained muscles, while it revitalizes and tones the body. The following suggestions for massage and for correcting posture will help the *victim type* to feel a new sense of pleasure and support in her body, and enable her to combat the stress and pressure of everyday life.

BALANCE THE BODY

ENCOURAGING FEELINGS of openness, strength, and stability, this exercise can be used on its own or when your partner stands up after a full massage. Softly guide these inner movements of energy with your hands, and use verbal imagery to help her become aware of, rather than force, changes in her posture.

MASSAGING TENSION AREAS

SPEND EXTRA TIME on aligning the body and give a feeling of length to the torso. Start with the massage sequence on pages 40-41.

THE TORSO

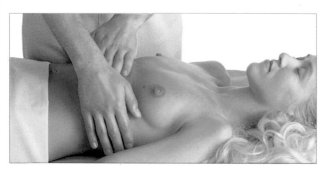

Relax chest and abdomen to deepen breathing and uncover underlying feelings. Use strokes to open, expand and soothe tension from the chest, diaphragm and abdomen (see pages 72-77).

ARMS AND HANDS

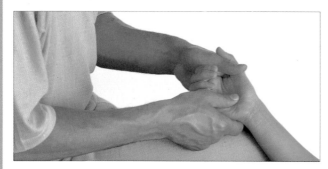

When the torso is more relaxed, connect the chest and arms with integrating strokes (see page 63). Massage and knead well into the arms to increase vitality, then work into the hands.

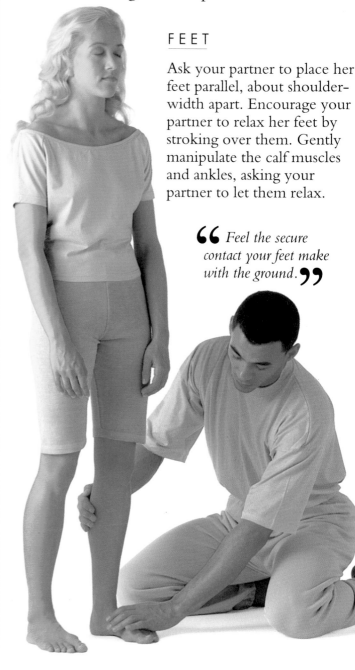

FEET

Ask your partner to place her feet parallel, about shoulder-width apart. Encourage your partner to relax her feet by stroking over them. Gently manipulate the calf muscles and ankles, asking your partner to let them relax.

❝ *Feel the secure contact your feet make with the ground.* **❞**

KNEES

Helping your partner to unlock her knees allows tension to be released from this vital area of the body. Gently place your hands over the knees and encourage your partner to loosen and relax them. When you feel the knees respond, stroke your hands down the legs to direct the release of tension down and out of the body.

PELVIS AND BUTTOCKS

Place your hands gently but firmly over the lower belly and base of the spine. Ask your partner to breathe into and relax this area. To encourage her pelvis to tuck under slightly and support her torso, ask her to imagine she has a heavy tail attached to the bottom of her spine which she releases and lets fall to the ground. Stroke your hands down from the pelvis, over the buttocks and down the legs.

❝ Let the tension and weight in your buttock muscles drop down toward the ground. ❞

❝Gently unlock your knees. ❞

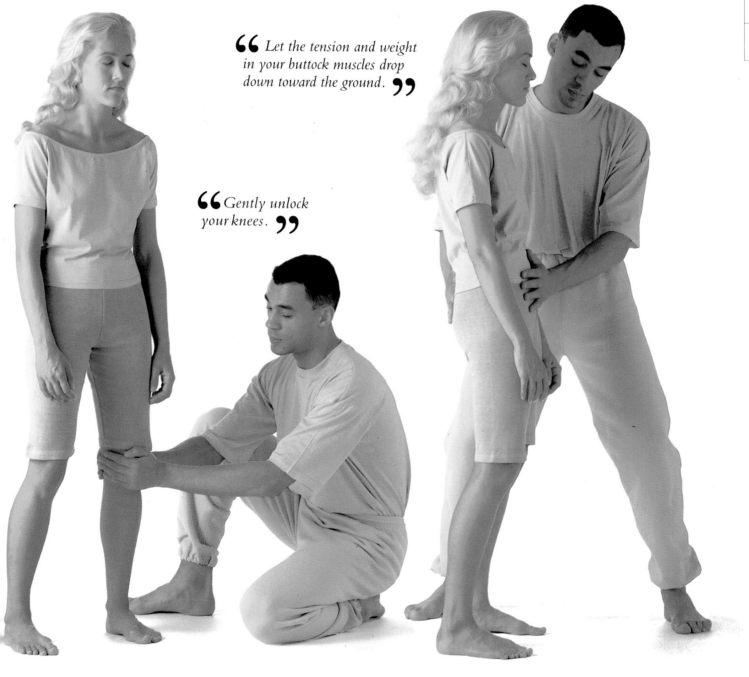

GROWING UPWARD

SECURELY SUPPORTED by her relaxed lower body and the ground beneath her feet, your partner will now be able to extend her spine and torso upward, giving her body a sense of length and grace and a reassuring feeling of "backbone". Then to increase the feeling of widening, opening up and expanding the body, so essential for a relaxed posture, encourage your partner to release tension locked in the back, chest, shoulders, and arms.

SPINE AND TORSO

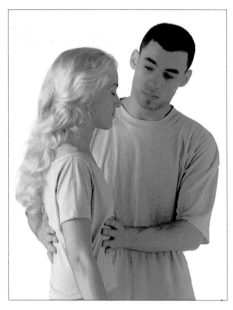

Glide your hands slowly up the front and back of the body. Ask her to breathe softly but deeply and feel a sense of extension as her torso lifts and her spine lengthens.

NECK AND HEAD

1 Having stroked up the torso, stop at the neck. Ask her to release up from the shoulders. Draw a hand up over the back of the neck and remind her to bring it in line with the spine.

2 As your hand reaches the △ base of your partner's skull, ask her to imagine that her head is floating up and away from her neck and spine. Ask her to feel a space between her neck and the base of her skull.

> *Imagine your head is a balloon floating up. Think of your spine as its string.*

3 Draw your hand up and over your partner's head. Gently pull upward on the hair at the top of her head. Ask her to feel support in her lower body as she allows her upper body to lengthen upward.

CHEST AND SHOULDER

Place your hands at the center of the body on the upper chest and back. Draw them slowly out toward the shoulder closest to you. Ask your partner to let this area widen and extend outward as if it were a bird's wing opening. Remind your partner to allow, not force, change in the body as she breathes fully and gently into the releasing areas.

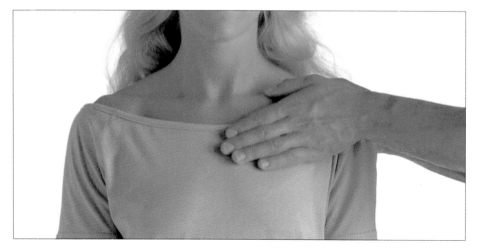

The breathing increases as the chest widens

ARM RELEASE

As the chest and shoulders widen, continue the movement from the shoulder joint down the arm, stopping to rock the elbow and wrist between your hands. Glide your hands down and out of your partner's hand and fingers.

" *Feel your arm lengthening down from the shoulder.* **"**

KEEPING THE BODY ALIGNED

Repeat the movements for the chest, shoulder, and arm on the other side of the body. Then return to any parts of the body that may still need realigning. Ask your partner to describe the changes she feels in her body, posture, breathing, and her emotions. Finally, encourage her to move around feeling a sense of stability, length, and width. Remind her to walk as if her head is floating upward, while the weight of her pelvis and her buttocks drops toward the ground.

EXTENDING THE SPINE

Deep massage strokes over the long spinal muscles focus your partner's awareness onto this crucial area of the body, release habitual strain and increase flexibility. At the same time, they lengthen the spine, and relax the neck and shoulder muscles. In this sequence, let your partner sit on a stool so she can lean forward under your strokes, enabling a deeper stretch.

Keep your shoulders relaxed

Extend your elbows to keep up the pressure

Use the flat edge of your knuckles

Lean forward slowly under the stroke

Stand so you can reach down the length of your partner's back comfortably

1 Make soft, relaxed fists and place your knuckles at the top of the back on each side of the spine. Slowly draw your knuckles down your partner's neck and out over her shoulders. ◁

2 Stretch the long muscles that run down the spine by placing your knuckles directly under the skull. Then draw them slowly and steadily down either side of the spine.

3 As you pull your fists down, your partner bends forward to encourage the depth and direction of your stroke. Continue down either side of your partner's spine. Do not run your knuckles over the spinal column itself. ▷

4 Finish your stroke at the base of the spine by gently releasing pressure. Repeat the sequence twice more, gradually increasing the pressure of the stroke.

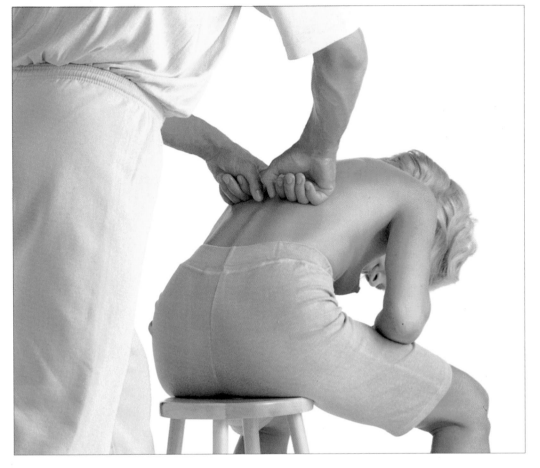

5 Ask your partner to bring her awareness to the alignment of her spine, neck and head by rolling her body slowly upward, vertebra by vertebra. Remind her to start at the bottom of the spine and roll up until her head balances above her spinal column. Focus her awareness onto her extended back by feather stroking (see page 121) up its full length.

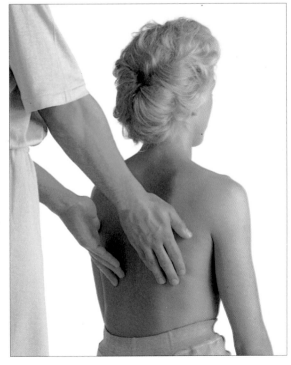

FINISHING TOUCHES

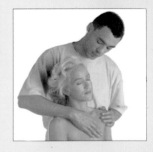

Having gently restored good posture, encourage your partner to rest back into the support of your body as she breathes fully and experiences a deep sense of relaxation.

*Letting go into deep
relaxation and refreshing
sleep is the gift that follows
a full and vibrant day.*

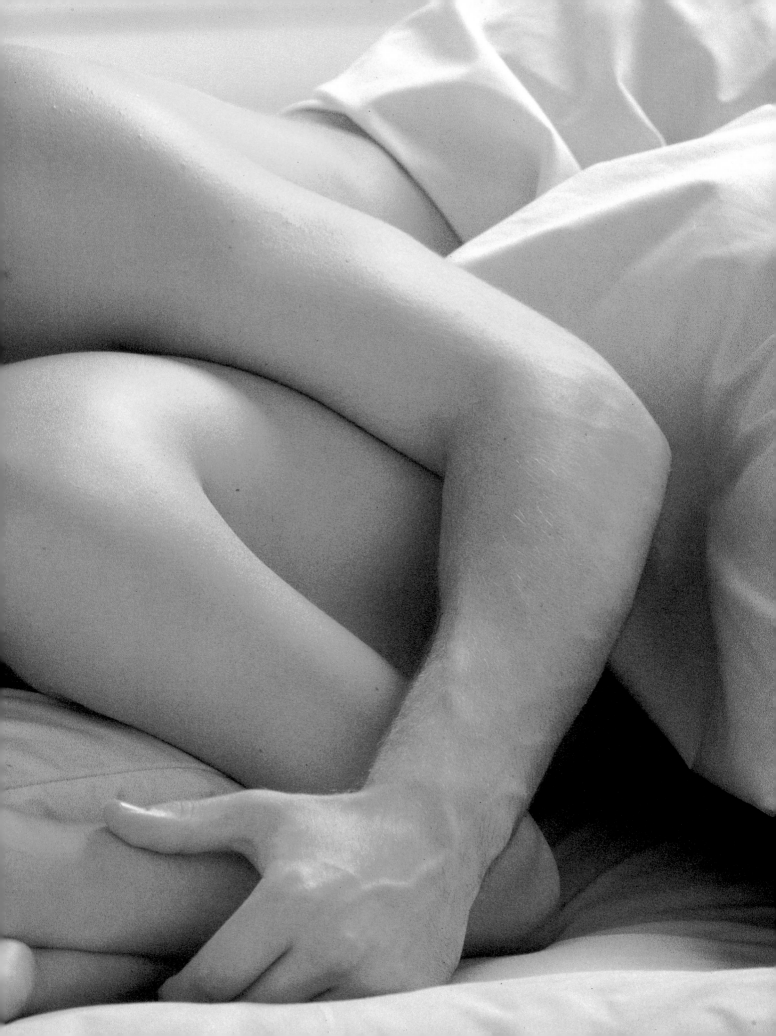

THE WARRIOR
A · PROGRAM · FOR · RELAXATION

The lift and release sequences are a series of deeply effective passive movements. They can help your partner trust you with his body, a factor vital for relaxation. By taking charge of the movements and supporting your partner's weight, you encourage him to release tension, and relax his control over his body. Introduce the movements after your partner has received several full massages and is beginning to relax, or use them as a session in themselves. Talk to your partner to encourage his relaxation and breathing (see page 35) or use the movements without verbal instructions in a full body massage. Work down both sides of his body.

HEAD AND NECK

TAKE THE WEIGHT of your partner's head and guide all the head's movements to help ease tension in the neck and under the ridge of the skull.

1 Stand behind your partner's head. Slide your hands under the skull and securely cup the head. Rest your middle fingers in the hollow at the top of the spine, thumbs on each side of the ears.

2 Ask your partner to drop the weight of his head into your hands, letting you do all the lifting and moving. Lift the head slowly and stretch the back of the neck as far as you both feel comfortable. ▽

3 Make sure that the head is in line with the spine as you gently lift and lower it several times. Continue to urge your partner to drop the heavy weight of his head back into the support of your hands.

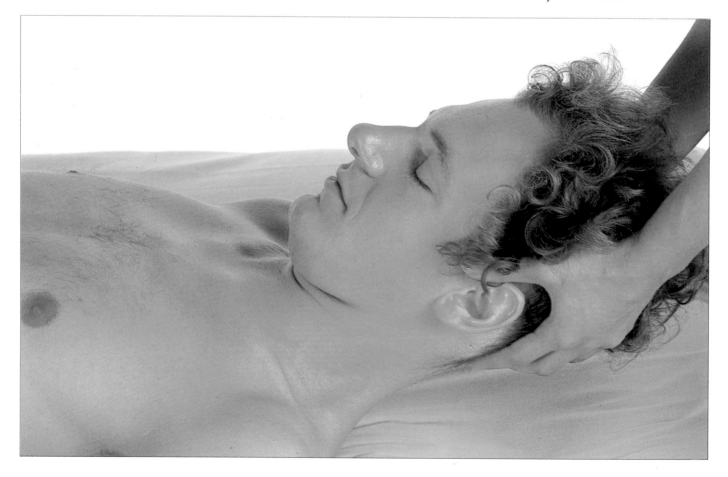

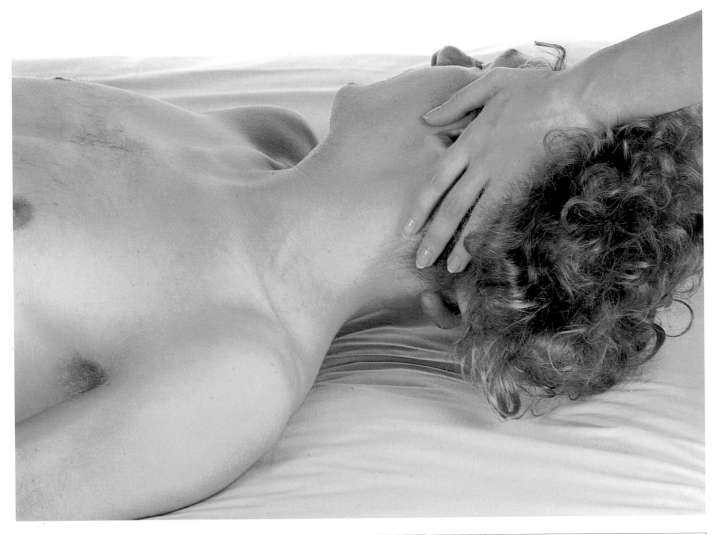

4 Turn the head slowly to △ rest in the left palm. Support it with the right hand on the other side. Lift slightly and roll the head to rest in your right palm. Roll the head several times.

5 Align your partner's head with his spine and rest it on the ridge of the skull. If the head continues to pull back, place a thin cushion or book, here covered with a towel, under it. ▷

6 Place your hands on each side of the forehead, thumbs over the center of the brow. Hold for some moments. Draw steadily up and out of the scalp.

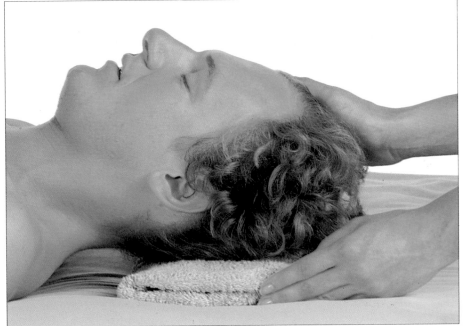

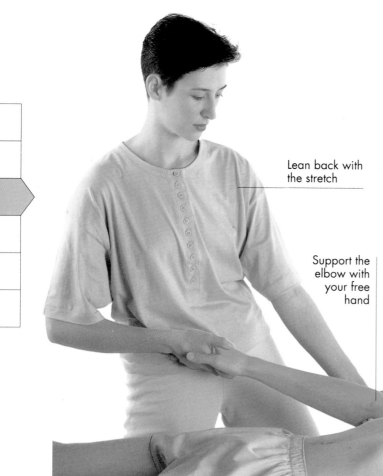

Lean back with
the stretch

Support the
elbow with
your free
hand

RELAXING THE JOINTS

LIFTING AND RELEASING the shoulders and arms
eases tension in the shoulder joints, helping
your partner breathe more freely into his
chest, and increasing his sense of relaxation.

1 Standing by your
partner's right side,
take his palm in your
right hand. With your
left hand, support his
slightly flexed elbow.
Position yourself to pull
the arm gently toward
you. Release slowly. ◁

2 Slowly lift the arm.
If your partner tries
to raise it for you, lower
the arm a little and ask
him to drop its weight
down into your hands.
Lift and lower until the
arm relaxes and grows
heavier in your hands.

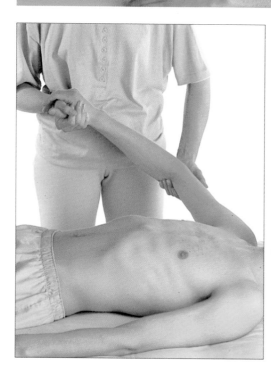

3 Keep your partner's
elbow flexed while
swinging his arm slightly
outward. Gently lift and
lower his arm from this
position.   ◁

4 Let go of the elbow
and clasp the wrist
between both hands. Lift
the arm upright to pull
gently on the shoulder
joint. As you lower the
arm slowly, support the
elbow with one hand to
keep it slightly flexed.
Place the arm back on
the mattress gently. ▷

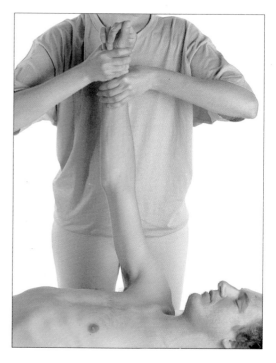

5 Clasp the wrist with your right hand and lift the arm up slightly, elbow flexed. Place your left hand behind the shoulder. Move yourself and the arm so it falls back into your left arm and hand, and rests above the head. ▷

6 Take the wrist and move so that you can place your left arm under the arm to support it. Lift the arm up and out in an arc back to the side of the body. Gently lower it.

Step back with the movement

Keep the elbow slightly flexed

Support the shoulder with your left hand

LOWER BACK AND PELVIS

SOOTHE LOWER BACK TENSION by encouraging your partner to drop his body into the support of your hands and the mattress.

At your partner's right side, slide your left hand under the lower back. Ask him to imagine the pelvis melting into your hand. Place your right hand over the abdomen. Ask your partner to relax as he exhales.

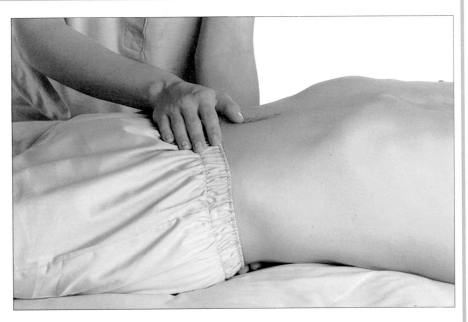

HIPS AND LEGS

A LOCKED-BACK PELVIS and rigid posture may cause tense hip joints and stiff legs. Loosen and relax them with the gentle lifting and releasing movements below. The legs may be heavy, so look after your own posture as you lift to prevent strains.

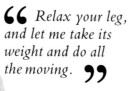

Relax your leg, and let me take its weight and do all the moving.

1 Stand by the lower leg on your partner's right side. Place your right hand under the heel from inside the foot, your left hand under the knee. Flex the knee slightly by pushing up from the heel. Lift and lower the leg slowly until it is heavier and looser. Gently swing the leg outward and back.

2 Move to stand at the bottom of the foot and clasp it firmly in both hands. Pull steadily toward you to create a gentle stretch in the hip and groin. Then slowly release the stretch. ▷

3 When you have relaxed both sides of the body, complete the session by placing the palms of your hands over the soles of both feet for some minutes while your partner rests.

Lean back with the stretch

Breathe steadily with the stretch and release

Pull the leg gently toward you

CHEST & ARM MASSAGE

Devote special attention to the braced shoulders,
inflated chest, and stiff arms of the *warrior type* during
a massage. As you soothe your partner's tense upper
body with a sequence of massage strokes that
connects his chest, arms and shoulders to each other,
you will deepen his sense of integration and
harmony in his body. The relaxing massage will also
release tension and increase flexibility.

SOOTHING THE CHEST AND ARMS

1 Stand by your partner's right side and place your
left hand behind the neck. Keeping your elbow
flexed, place your right hand over the base of your
partner's breastbone. Slide your right hand steadily
upward, using pressure from your fingertips, and
simultaneously draw your left hand down to
rest behind the shoulder.

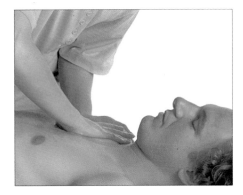

Keep your
elbow flexed

Encourage
your partner
to breathe
into the stroke

2 At the top of the breastbone,
swing your right hand toward
the shoulder, applying pressure
with the heel of your hand.

3 When both your hands are
holding the shoulder, change
your position to pull firmly down
both sides of your partner's arm
and out of the fingers. Repeat the
sequence on the opposite side.

A thin book (covered
here by a towel) helps
to create space at the
base of the skull

ARM MASSAGE

FURTHER HELP THE RELEASE of tension from the shoulder joint with lift and release movements (see pages 60-61). Then use these deeper tissue strokes and spreading stretch movements to release tightness in the arms.

UPPER ARM RELEASE

Support the shoulder with your left hand. Make a fist with the right hand and place it on the muscle below the shoulder. Sink down with the flat area between the knuckles and finger joints. When the muscle relaxes, slowly draw down over it. ▽

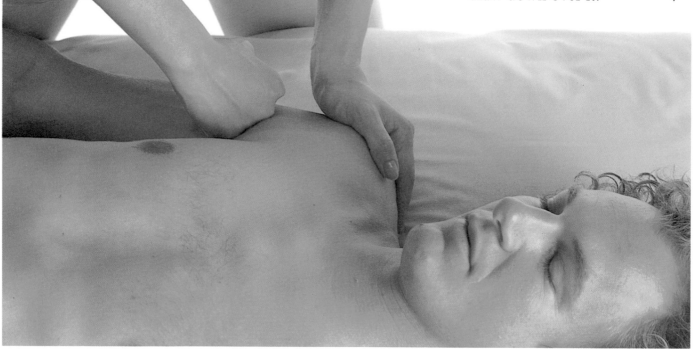

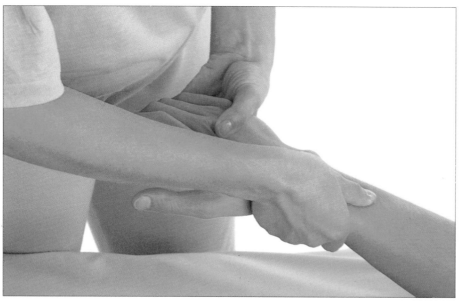

MUSCLE STRETCH

Slip your fingers under the upper arm to support it. Place the heels of your hands in the center of the arm. Slide firmly outward and down toward the mattress. Continue down to the wrist.

LOWER ARM RELEASE

Lift your partner's hand up slightly. Sink the thumb on your right hand into the furrow between the two long bones at the center of the wrist. Slide slowly up the arm to the outside of the elbow. ◁

WRISTS AND HANDS

THE SMALL, SLIDING WRIST bones give the
hands mobility, which is diminished when
the arms are stiff or the hands are held
clenched. To relax the wrist, try these
joint release movements, then add strokes
to stretch and relieve tension in
the intricate network of bones and
muscles of the hands.

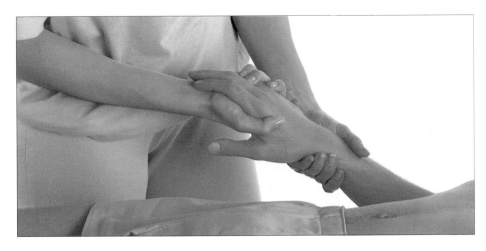

FLEXING THE WRIST

Support the arm and take your
partner's hand. First flex the wrist
up and down, then turn the joint
from side to side. Repeat these
movements several times.

RELAXING THE HANDS

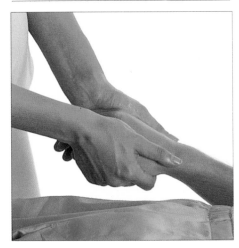

1 Support the palm with your
fingers. Draw the heels of your
hands and your thumbs across the
back of the hand from the center
outward. Move down from the
wrist to the knuckles.

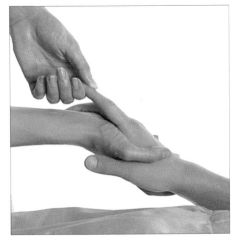

2 Hold the hand, palm down
in your right hand. Stretch
each finger, gently pulling from
the base to the tip with your left
thumb and index finger. Change
hands to stretch the thumb.

FINISHING TOUCHES

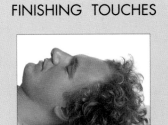

Allow your partner time
to rest and assimilate the
effects of the massage.
Then add to his sense
of relaxation by gently
holding his hand, and
resting your other hand
over his heart.

THE INTELLECTUAL
A · PROGRAM · FOR · RELAXATION

Draw energy away from the head and mind, back down into the body, with a whole body massage. Your soft touches will also encourage natural vitality that has contracted inside your partner to expand outward, helping to release deep-seated tension. As your partner senses the different parts of her body becoming more integrated, she will feel more comfortable. The calming holds that follow can be included in a massage to induce further relaxation.

MASSAGING TENSION AREAS

ENCOURAGE YOUR PARTNER to breathe into tense areas of her body as you massage them. Always be gentle and accepting while giving a massage: your partner will only retreat into her tension if she feels criticized.

JOINT AREAS

Massage thoroughly into the tense shoulders, neck, and head (see pages 103–107). ▷

RELEASING STROKES

Massage to draw energy down the body, and always direct tension out of the extremities: the arms, legs, head and neck (see hand stroking page 121).

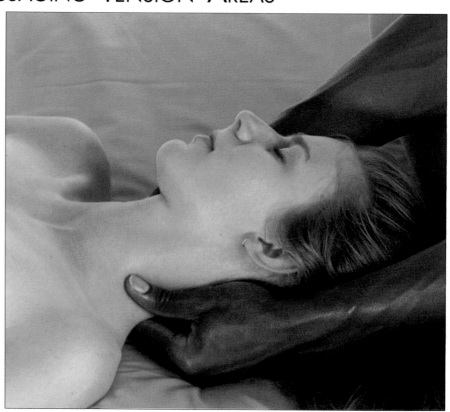

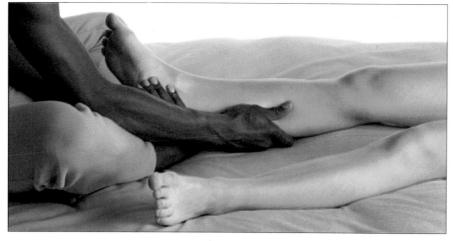

LEGS AND FEET

As your partner begins to enjoy and relax into the massage, spend extra time on the feet, ankles, and legs (see pages 98–101). Once she is more familiar with this part of the body, you can start to increase the pressure of your strokes. ◁

RESTORING BALANCE

RELAXING HOLDS THAT CONNECT different parts of your partner's body will have a particularly calming effect, promoting restful feelings of harmony and equilibrium. Start these soothing connection holds with your partner lying on her back, either undressed or lightly clothed, and follow a flowing sequence around both sides of the body, moving from top to bottom. Always approach the body and withdraw your hands gently and slowly, and to deepen the meditative effect of each hold, stay aware of your own relaxed body and breathing.

HEAD HOLD

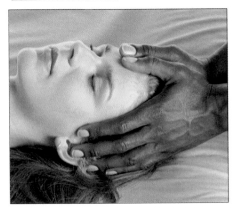

Clasp the head, with your fingers placed symmetrically on each side of the scalp, thumbs resting over the center of the forehead. When ready, slowly draw your hands out through the hair.

HEAD-NECK

Place your left hand over the forehead, fingers pointing to the right side of the head. Place your right hand behind the neck, fingers pointing toward the left side. Release when ready.

HEAD-HEART

Rest your left hand against the side of the head, thumb over the center of your partner's brow. Place your right hand over the heart. Ask your partner to focus on her breathing and on the area between your hands. ▷

Close
your eyes

Allow your
breath to flow
deep into your
abdomen

Encourage your
partner to breathe
into your hands

Exhale into
your hands

SHOULDER-HAND

1 Place your left hand behind your partner's right shoulder. Take her hand. Imagine breathing warmth into the area of the body between your hands. ▷

2 Release the shoulder and stroke down past the elbow. Now connect the elbow and hand.

"Focus your awareness on the parts of your body beneath my hands. Breathe into them."

Holding your partner's hand is very comforting for her

Close your eyes

HAND-HEART

Still holding the right hand, rest the left hand gently on the heart.

HEART-ABDOMEN

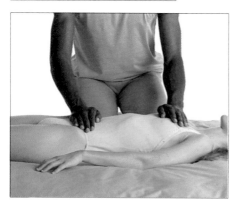

Keeping your hand over the heart, move your right hand slowly to rest below the navel. Encourage your partner to let her breath meet your hands.

HIP-FOOT

1 To bring relaxation and warmth to the joints, place your left hand on your partner's right hip, your right hand over the knee. Release when ready.

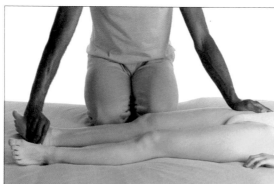

2 With your left hand on the hip, △ clasp the sole of the foot with your right hand. Imagine your breath passing through and relaxing your partner's leg. Stroke from above the hip to the foot.

THE FEET

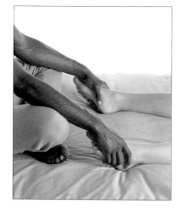

Hold your partner's foot between your hands. Place your right hand over the left foot and hold both feet to bring balance to both sides of the body. Repeat all the holds on this page on your partner's left side.

BALANCING THE BACK OF THE BODY

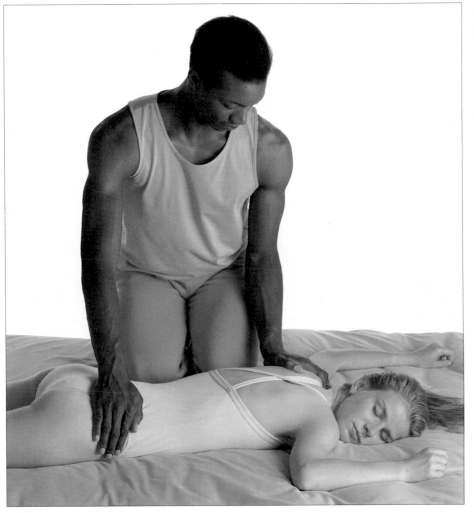

ASK YOUR PARTNER TO LIE on her front, and gently make soothing connection holds on both sides of the back of her body.

NECK-SACRUM

Place your hands at the top (the neck) and bottom (the sacrum) of the spine. Encourage your partner to focus her awareness on and breathe into your hands.

SHOULDER-HIP

Bring a balance to the left and right sides of the body by placing your left hand behind your partner's left shoulder, and your right hand over her right hip. ◁

SACRUM-FOOT

Place your left hand over the sacrum, your right hand over the sole of the left foot to connect the upper and lower halves of the body (below left).

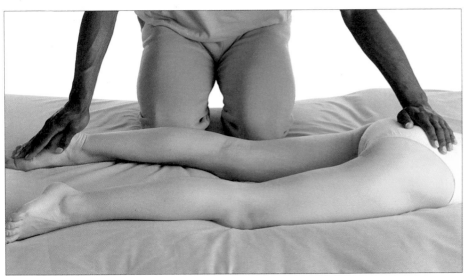

FINISHING TOUCHES

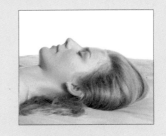

Ask your partner to turn onto her back and rest as she feels her body in harmony. Gently cover her with a sheet.

Touch is a language of love. Even the gentlest of caresses can convey a depth of feeling and help your partner shed the tension of the day.

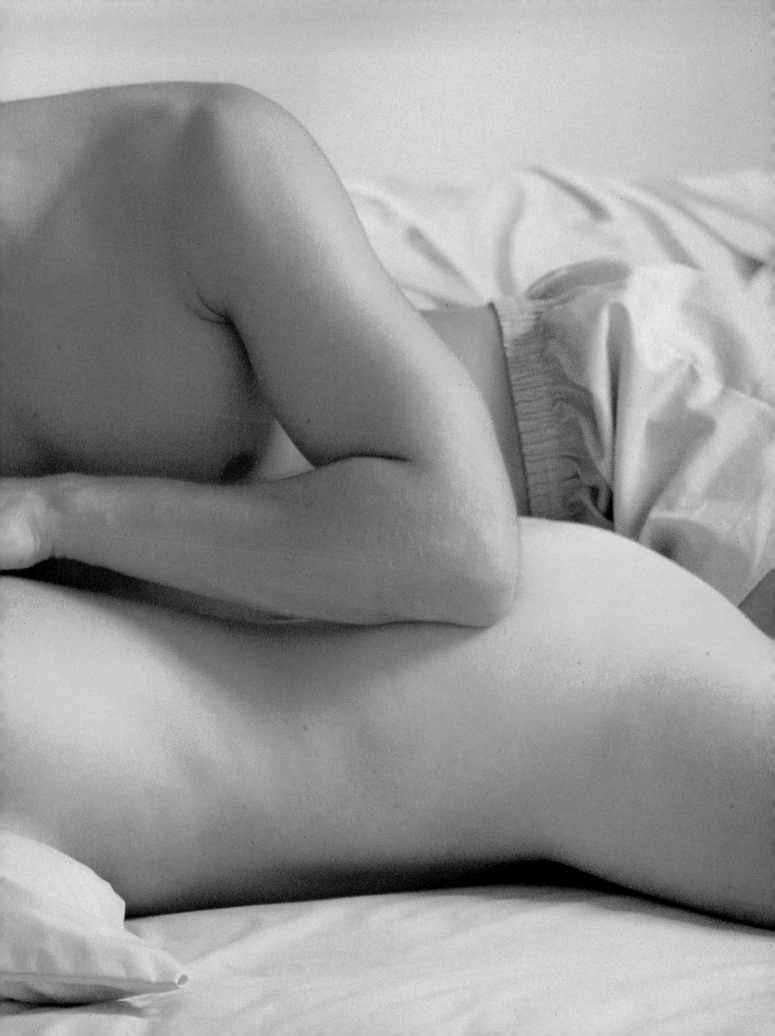

THE SUPERMAN
A · PROGRAM · FOR · RELAXATION

This sensitive massage sequence will help your partner relax, let go of his tough image, and allow his tensions to melt away. Gently calm the body with soft massage strokes before applying deeper pressure. Then, using the soothing strokes below, devote special attention to relaxing the abdomen and diaphragm, areas that easily become tense in the effort to suppress and control the powerful, instinctive emotions rooted there. When massaging this area, always approach it gently, and pause to give your partner time to relax. Start the sequence by smoothing a little oil or lotion on your hands, and rub them together to warm them.

ABDOMEN ROCK

Kneel on the mattress or stand beside your partner's hip and slide your hands under each side of the body just above the pelvis so your fingers touch the spine. Lift the area up slightly and rock it back and forth as your hands slide apart. When they reach the edge of the body allow the back to sink down onto the mattress. ▽

RELAXING HOLD

Position yourself by your partner's side. Slide one hand under the back, rest the other parallel to it just below the navel. Encourage your partner to breathe into the area between your hands and imagine the muscles softening. Withdraw your hands as he relaxes.

Keep your breath steady and flowing

Raise yourself up on one leg as you lift

CROSS-OVER STROKE

Take care of your back with this stroke. Do not try it if your partner is too heavy

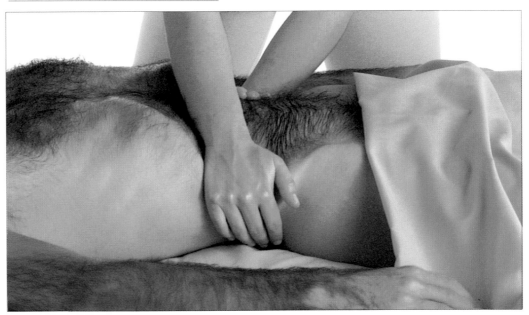

1 Place your hands over your partner's hips, making sure your fingers are pointing away from you. Then slowly slide your hands past each other to the opposite side of your partner's body, taking your stroke down toward the mattress beneath him.

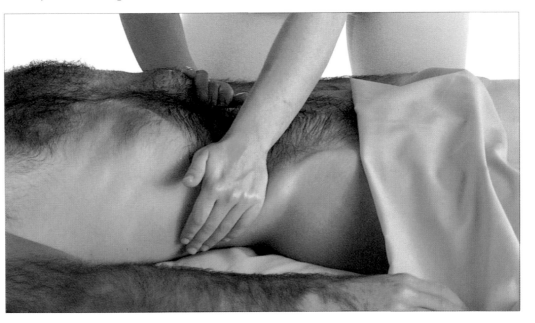

2 Without breaking the flow of this cross-over stroke, slide your hands back to their original position at the start of the stroke. Let your hands cross over your partner's body in a continuous motion, moving them up over his abdomen to the rib cage and then back again. Repeat the whole sequence several times up and down the body.

73

CIRCULAR STROKE

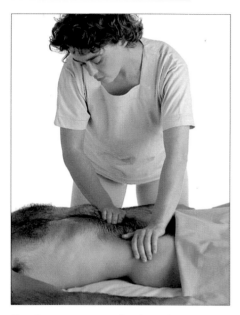

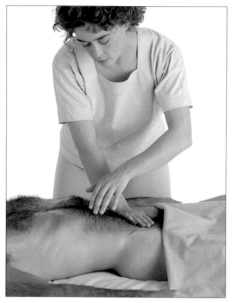

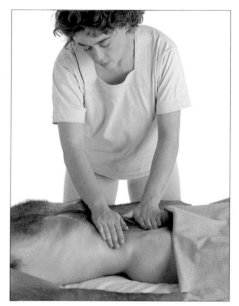

1 Place your right hand over the upper abdomen below the rib cage. Place your left hand over the lower abdomen. When your partner feels easy with your touch, slide your right hand clockwise around the abdomen.

2 Then lift up your lower, passive hand to allow the moving hand to pass it, as your moving hand makes a circle in a clockwise direction around your partner's entire upper and lower abdomen.

3 Then return your passive, lower hand to your partner's lower abdomen, making a crescent movement from one side of his pelvis to the other. Repeat this stroke several times.

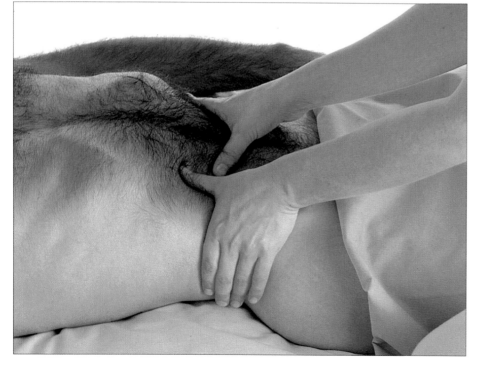

THUMB ROLLING

Place your thumbs one above the other at the bottom right side of the lower abdomen. Using short strokes, bring the top thumb back behind the other, pressing into the flesh so that they follow each other in an upward movement. Thumb roll in this way up over the upper and lower abdomen, working in small sections from right to left.

FLESH SCOOP

Make sure the skin is not too oily.
Then using your fingertips as a hook,
your thumbs as an anchor, scoop
up the flesh and muscle from
the center of the upper
abdomen and rock it
gently back and forth.
Release slowly.

Keep your back
straight and think
about your posture

Flex your
elbows slightly

Clasp the muscle
with fingertips
and thumbs

FREEING THE BREATH

Massaging around and under the rib cage helps to unlock tension in the diaphragm, which is essential for overall physical and emotional relaxation. As you relax the area, the breath will begin to flow more freely through your partner's body, like a wave rising and falling with each inhalation and exhalation. Pent-up feelings of fear, anxiety, and anger will release gently, as a refreshing sense of vitality and energy is restored.

ENCOURAGING BREATHING

1 Stand beside your partner's torso. Slip one hand under the back, at the base of the rib cage. Place the other over the solar plexus area, just below the breastbone. Ask your partner to breathe gently into the area between your hands, with emphasis on the out breath, and to imagine each breath melting tensions away.

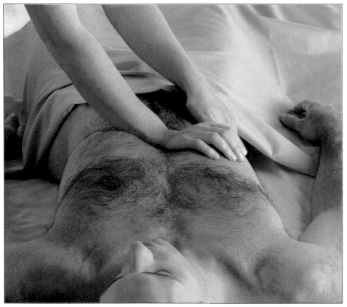

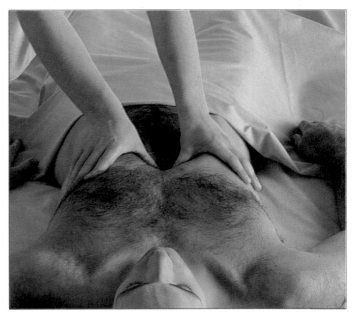

2 Massage thoroughly into the area below your partner's breastbone and the base of his rib cage by making rotary motions with the heel of your hand. Keep your elbow flexed and your arm relaxed throughout. Add a little pressure to your stroke as your partner relaxes, but always remain sensitive to his responses.

3 Now use your thumbs to stretch and release the muscle beneath the rib cage. Place your hands on each side of the rib cage, thumbs resting just under the breastbone. Draw your thumbs down under the base of the rib cage, sinking gently but fully into the muscle under the ribs. Repeat this stroke three times.

HEART-ABDOMEN HOLD

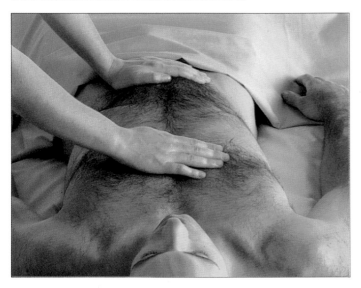

Place your right hand over the heart area, and your left hand on your partner's abdomen. Let the warmth and touch of your hands continue to melt away your partner's tensions.

FINISHING TOUCHES

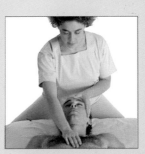

A soothing hold that connects your partner's head and heart will allow him gently to assimilate the changes taking place in his body and his emotions as he relaxes after the massage session.

THE STOIC
A · PROGRAM · FOR · RELAXATION

Massage strokes that bring length and lightness to the body, and increase the feeling of extending upward against the pull of gravity, are ideal for relaxing someone with a *stoic type* body. To release back tension, start by using relaxing strokes over the entire back, with your partner lying on her front. Work into tense, tight muscles around the neck and shoulders. Kneading strokes, or strokes using the thumbs and fingertips (see pages 122-23), are particularly effective when massaging into these muscles. The deeper strokes that follow should be applied with sensitivity (see page 35) to both sides of the body.

PALPITATION

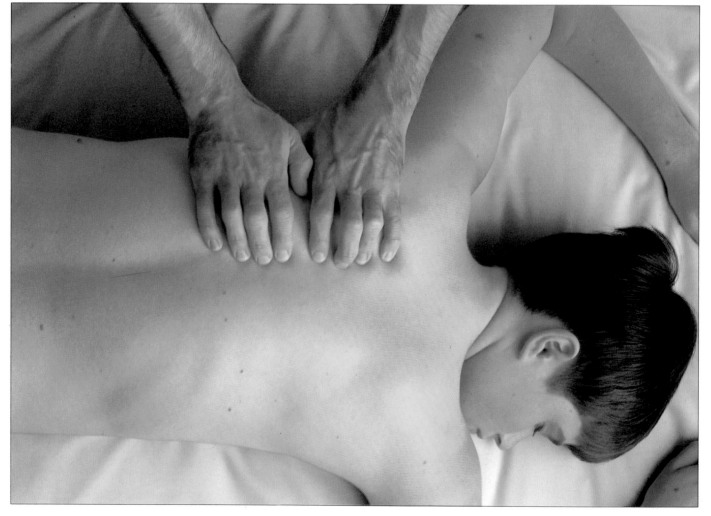

To prepare the area for a deeper stretch stroke, hook your fingertips (knuckles slightly bent, hands relaxed) into the area immediately along one side of the vertebrae at the top of your partner's spine. Create a slight rocking motion with your fingers. Continue this palpitation movement down alongside the spine.

LONG STRETCH

1 Stand by your partner's shoulder. Place the flat of your elbow and broad surface of the forearm on the area between the top of the shoulder blade and the spine. Move to face the stroke and lean your weight into the arm. Sink your arm to the right depth for the stroke (see page 35) and ask your partner to focus her awareness on the stroke and breathe into it. Slowly and steadily move down the back. ▽

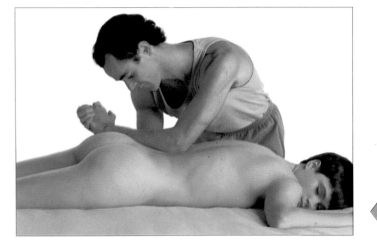

2 As your hand and wrist pass over the lower back onto the buttocks, swing them toward you at a 45° angle and slide your stroke more lightly over the pelvis and buttocks, out toward the hip.

Clasp your working hand with your free hand to add support

Lean into your stroke

Use the broad surface of your arm and the flat of the elbow

DEEPER STROKES

Relax the lower back, pelvis, and buttocks with deeper massage strokes to unlock emotional tension rooted in the muscles. First massage the whole area with soothing strokes (see page 120), then slowly stretch and ease muscles in the buttocks and thighs with the strokes below. Loosen tight calves during your massage, first by relaxing them with gentle strokes, then by kneading well into the muscles with the tips of your thumbs (see page 122). Stretch strokes will also help to release tension from painful calves.

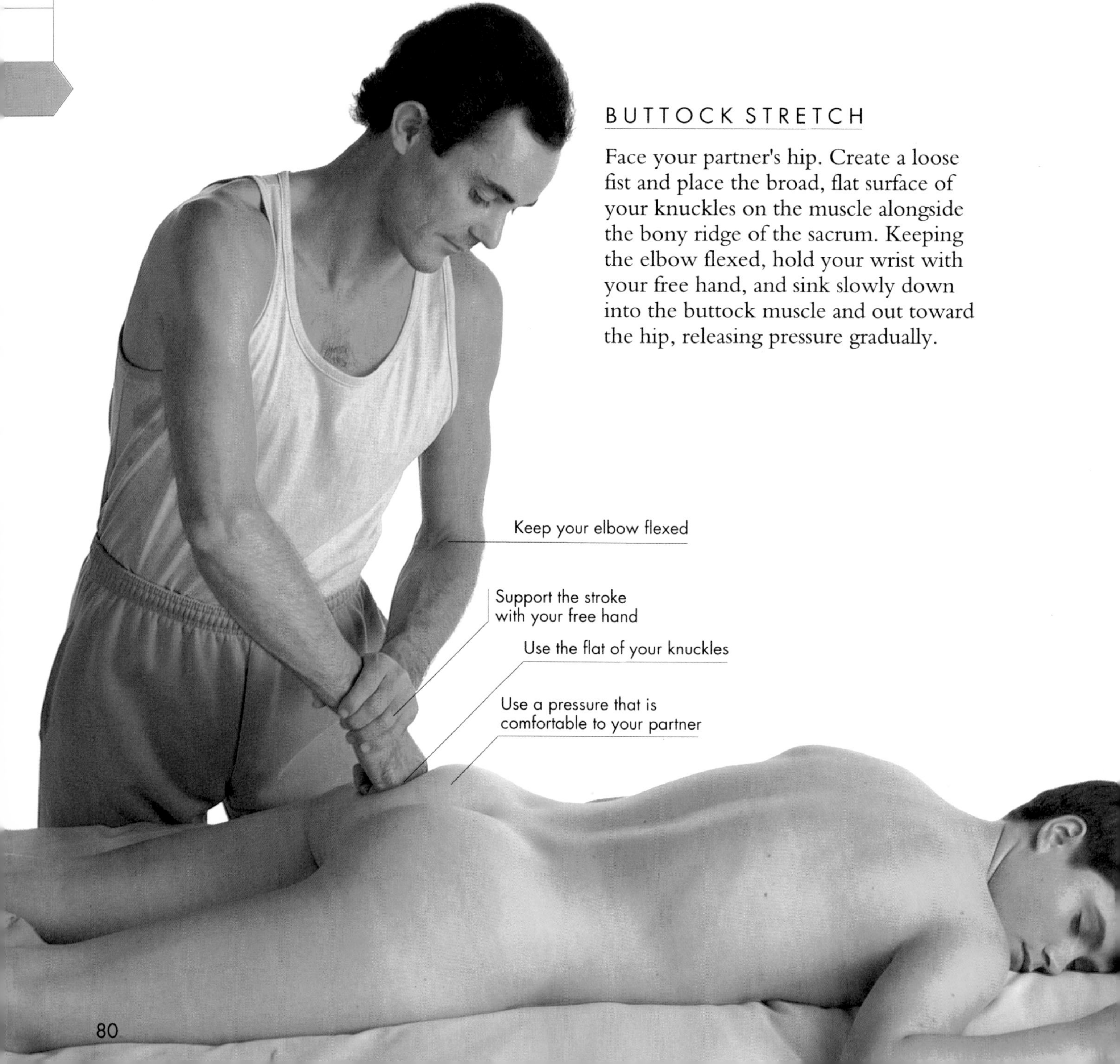

BUTTOCK STRETCH

Face your partner's hip. Create a loose fist and place the broad, flat surface of your knuckles on the muscle alongside the bony ridge of the sacrum. Keeping the elbow flexed, hold your wrist with your free hand, and sink slowly down into the buttock muscle and out toward the hip, releasing pressure gradually.

Keep your elbow flexed

Support the stroke with your free hand

Use the flat of your knuckles

Use a pressure that is comfortable to your partner

LONG THIGH STRETCH

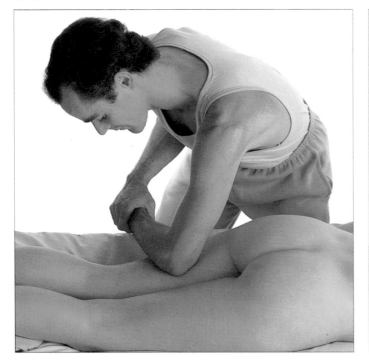

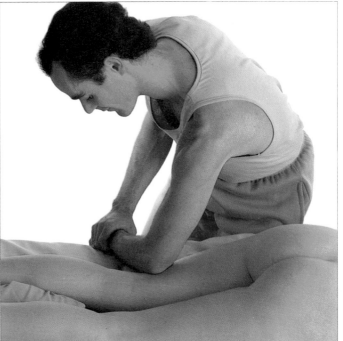

1 Standing by the thigh, place your elbow and forearm at an angle on the buttocks and position yourself to lean into the stroke. Using the flat of the elbow, not the edge, hook the surface of your arm into the muscle and slowly slide down the thigh.

2 Feel the thigh muscle lengthen and release. As your hand and wrist approach the back of the knee, lighten the pressure and swing out of the leg. Never apply pressure to the delicate and sensitive area of the back of the knee.

SQUEEZING THE MUSCLE

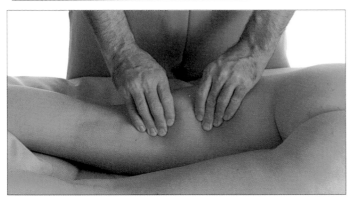

STRETCHING THE CALVES

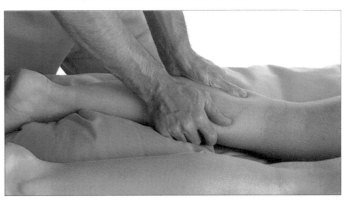

Hook the muscle on the back of the thigh with your fingertips. Anchor the hold with your thumbs and pull the flesh toward you. Squeeze it gently, and rock the flesh back and forth between your fingers and thumbs for some moments. You may also use this movement on the calves.

Place the heels of your hands in the center of the calf, fingers gripping the front of the leg, thumbs pointing up the back of the leg. Slide the heels firmly out toward the side of the leg. Move down the calf and then repeat the stroke.

ANKLES AND FEET

LOOSEN TIGHT, TENSE ANKLES with the following movements to increase mobility and relax the joints. Then gently but firmly create a slow, smooth stretch through the feet to relieve the tension and help them provide a comfortable, stable support for your partner's body weight.

SHAKING THE ANKLE

Lift the lower leg so that the knee is bent. Clasp the leg just below the ankle and shake it rhythmically to set up a rocking motion through the foot and ankle joint, and down through the calf muscles.

Rock the ankle

Clasp the leg between both hands

The rocking creates a wave of movement through the leg

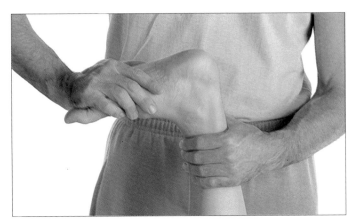

TENDON STRETCH

To stretch the tendons at the back of the ankle, hold the ankle from behind with your left hand, place your right hand over the sole, and gently push downward. Slowly ease the pressure to relax the stretch.

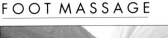

FOOT MASSAGE

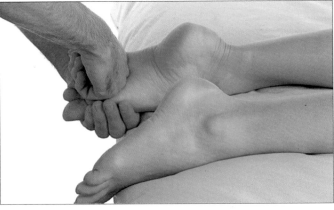

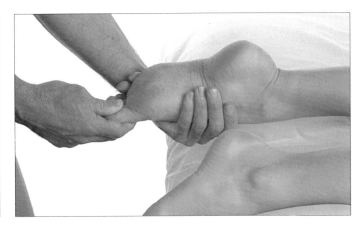

1 Clasp the foot in your left hand while placing the broad flat edge of the knuckles on your right hand into the heel. Apply pressure, pulling down firmly over the surface of the sole and the ball of the foot to the base of the toes.

2 Swap hands, then clasp each toe in turn at its base between thumb and forefinger. Stretch-pull down to its tip. Change the position of your hands again to stretch the big toe.

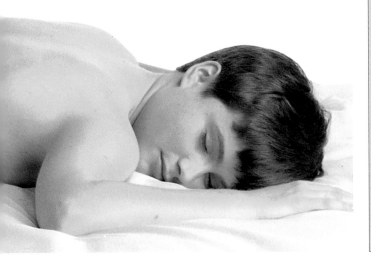

FINISHING TOUCHES

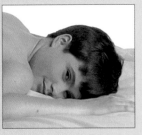

At the end of the massage clasp your partner's feet. Shake them rhythmically to send a wave of movement through her body. To induce deeper relaxation, hold the feet for a while.

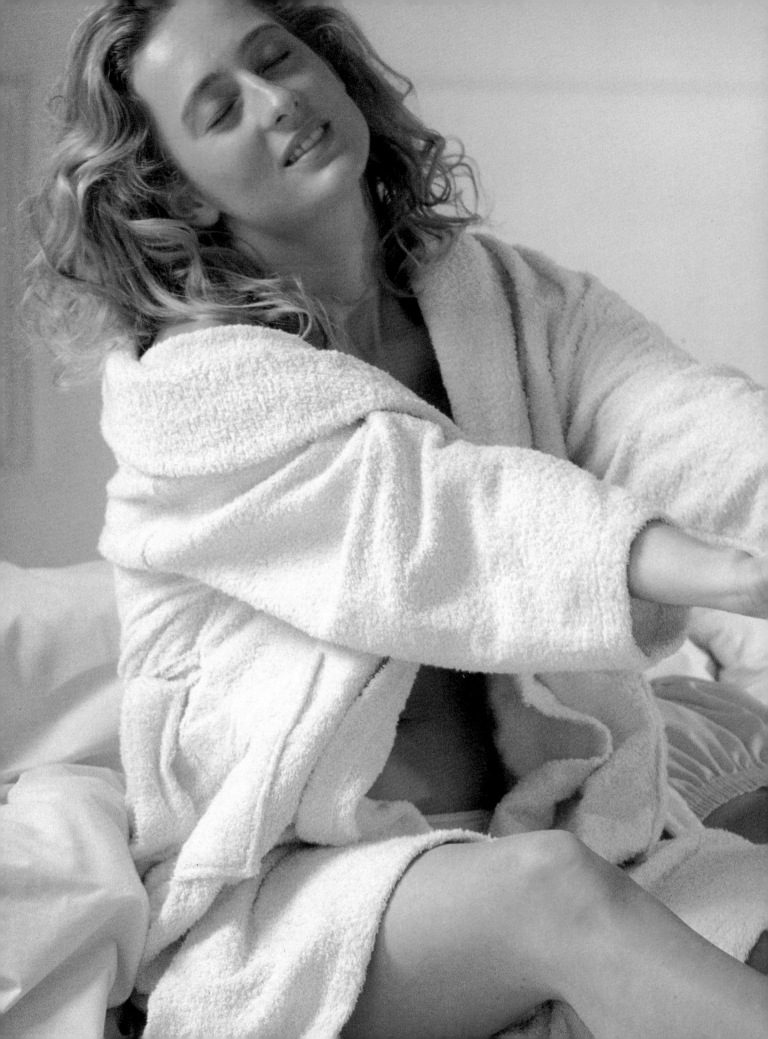

4
RELIEVING WORK-RELATED STRESS

Ease away the pain, headaches and back problems associated with day to day stress and work conditions through massage. These programs soothe and replenish those in different jobs, from the executive who finds it hard to unwind, to people in more physically demanding work. Also included is a self-massage sequence, suitable for all occupations.

EXECUTIVE STRESS
RELAXING · THE · OVERTIRED · MIND

When faced with the pressures of the work-place, it is essential to find a balance between work and rest. The perfect antidote to stress, massage can help to do this. Even a fifteen-minute massage on the neck, head and face at the end of a hectic day eases tension and revitalizes the body. A massage also helps the mind to switch off after an anxious day. Combine the massage ideas below with the strokes on pages 106-107, focusing on tension spots at the base of the neck, jaw, temples, brow and forehead.

KNEADING THE BASE OF THE NECK

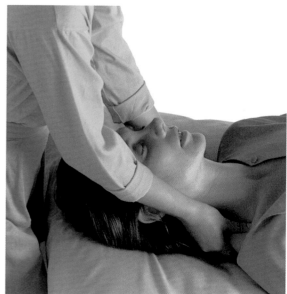

Kneading alleviates the tightness in the base of the neck that causes headaches by restricting circulation. Start by anchoring your thumbs over the top of the shoulders and slide your fingers down the back. Then, alternating hands, rhythmically and steadily knead the muscles at the base of the neck and above the shoulder blades by scooping up the flesh with your fingertips, pulling it toward you, then releasing.

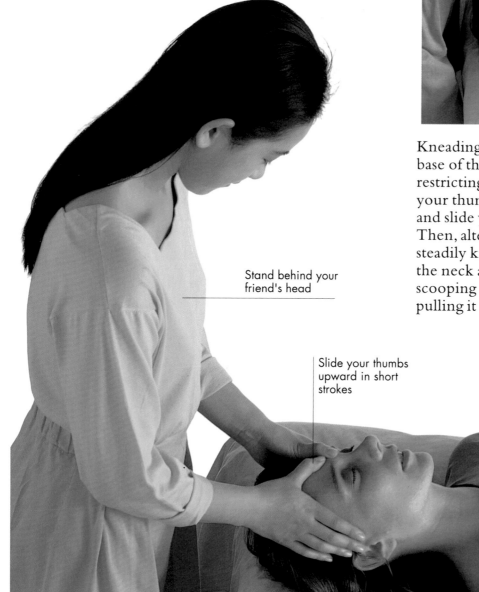

Stand behind your friend's head

Slide your thumbs upward in short strokes

EASING A TENSE FOREHEAD

Soothe away the worry and anxiety that furrow the muscles in the center of the brow. Place your thumbs between the eyebrows, and spread the muscles with short, upward-sliding strokes. ◁

RELAXING THE TEMPLES

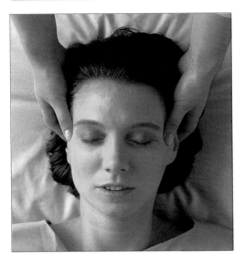

Stress can tighten the scalp and the temples, straining the muscles around the eyes. Soothe and relax this area by supporting the head between your hands. Then, making circular movements with your thumbs, firmly sweep around the temples several times until you feel them relaxing.

SOFTENING THE FACE MUSCLES

The warmth of your hands will soothe and soften the muscles of the face, and this is a wonderfully calming way to complete a face massage. First briskly rub your hands together to warm them. Then place your hands gently over your friend's eyes and cheeks for several moments.

EYEBROW PRESSURE POINT

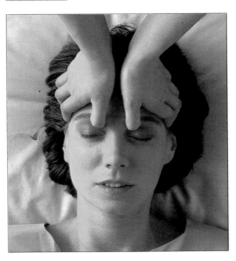

Use this thumb stroke to clear the mind and ease headaches. Sensitively and gradually press into the indentation of the bone just beneath the inside corner of both eyebrows. Add pressure slowly and carefully as this can be a painful movement. Release gently after several moments.

LOOSENING THE JAW

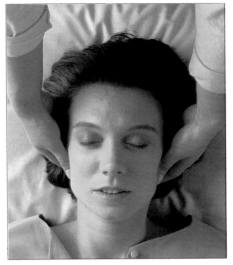

Place your index fingers under the jaw. Loosen the muscle over the jawbone with short sliding thumb strokes. Work from the center of the chin to the outer edge of the jaw. Then massage into the jaw joint with circular thumb motions. Add pressure gradually as the muscles relax.

THE RELAXED DRIVER

Getting stuck in a traffic jam, being overtaken by an aggressive driver, or crawling along on a congested road when you have an important appointment to keep are all likely to cause you maximum stress and anxiety. Driving is hard on body and mind, and it is important to feel calm to cope with the tensions that can arise from it. Start by playing soothing music on the cassette deck, keep breathing deeply, and take the time to relax your body consciously. Loosen the tight grip of your hands on the steering wheel, allow your shoulders to drop, and let your jaw and mouth soften. Always plan your route carefully, and give yourself plenty of time. Adjust your seat to allow you to sit upright with plenty of room for your legs when driving long distances. Stop every once in a while and take a walk to stretch the legs and boost circulation. When you arrive home, ask someone to give you a massage to rid your body of driving stress. The worst-affected areas are the shoulders, neck, and jaw. Use the strokes shown here to loosen a stiff neck and tight face muscles. The massage on pages 90-91 will also benefit drivers. Ease tense hands using the strokes on page 95.

PHYSICAL STRESS
RELAXING · THE · OVERWORKED · BODY

People in physically strenuous occupations are particularly prone to back injuries, usually in the lower or middle back. The majority of these injuries occur when bending, lifting, twisting unnecessarily or awkwardly, over-stretching, or moving stiff muscles suddenly. Prolonged repetitive movements with one part of the body also cause wear and tear on the joints. Using your body correctly and taking care of your back and posture helps you stay active both in and out of work. Stretching in the morning keeps the back muscles supple and prepares the spine for a day's work. Gentle massage at the end of the day brings great relief to tired, sore muscles, takes tension out of the spine, and restores your energy.

MOVING CORRECTLY

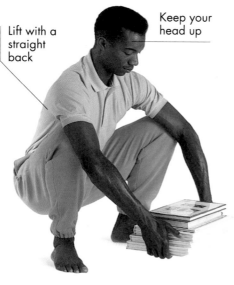

Lift with a straight back

Keep your head up

■ Do not twist when you are reaching or moving.
■ Always directly face your activity, and make sure your back is straight.
■ Keep work tools tidy and within reach to avoid over-stretching and unnecessary bending and pulling.
■ Avoid continuous repetitive movement in one part of the body. Take breaks, then do a different task.
■ Change your body position frequently to prevent stiffness.

■ If you have a persistent back pain, consult your doctor, and always check with a doctor before trying out any new exercises. If an exercise causes discomfort, stop at once.
■ When bending and lifting, keep your head up and your back straight while bending in the knees. Then push up using the large leg muscles. Do not lift anything that is too heavy for you (check the weight by lifting a corner), and hold the load close to your body.

RELAXING THE BODY

After an active day, take fifteen minutes to relax and refresh your whole body. Start by lying down on a firm mattress or on the floor. Consciously let the weight of your body sink down into the support beneath you. Breathe slowly and gently into each part of your body, letting it relax more deeply with every exhalation.

LOOSENING THE LOWER BACK

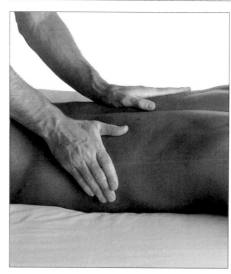

1 Massage the back with soft, flowing strokes, then use the strokes on pages 108-109.

2 Place your hands on each side of the base of the spine, fingers pointing upward. Make continuous alternate circles, adding pressure with the side of your thumbs, and heels. Work thoroughly on the lower back, then up to the shoulder blades. Sweep your hands up and over the shoulders to finish. ◁

SPINE RELEASE

Place both thumbs in the groove alongside the vertebrae at the base of the spine. Rest your hands and fingers at an angle facing away from the spine. Slide them firmly and steadily up each side of the spine. At the top, sweep over the shoulders, then glide your hands down the sides of the body and back to the source of your stroke. Repeat the sequence three times.

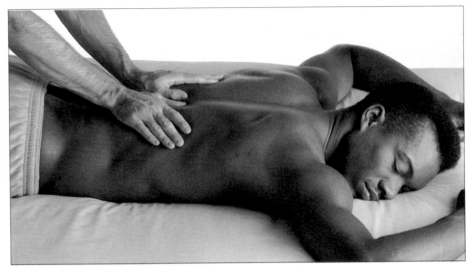

EXTENDING THE BACK

Lie down on your front. Rest your elbows at a right angle to your body to support it. Look forward and raise your head.

Stretch your head and neck back as far as possible. Hold the stretch, then lower yourself gradually to the floor. Repeat up to ten times.

FLEXING

Lie on your back. Bring your knees to your chest and clasp your hands over them. Round your head up toward your knees. Relax back to the floor, then repeat up to ten times.

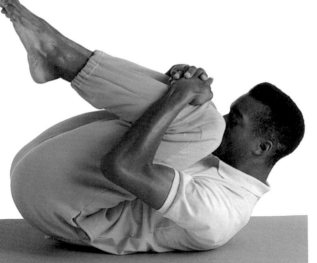

WORKING IN THE HOME

A little thought can prevent stress and strain. Do not stoop when picking up objects or talking to children: bend and lift as suggested. When vacuuming, keep your feet apart, your spine straight, and bend your knees. Do not overload yourself with shopping bags; distribute the weight evenly. If you carry a baby on your hip, change sides frequently. When gardening, kneel or sit on a low stool for weeding, and use the leg muscles when bending, lifting, or pulling.

SEDENTARY STRESS
RELAXING · THE · INACTIVE · BODY

The body is not designed for long periods of inactivity, and sedentary jobs, particularly if they involve sitting, studying and working at a desk, take their toll. When you slump, lean forward, concentrate intensely, and reduce your breath, tension accumulates around the spine and upper back. Sore shoulders and a stiff neck are the most common complaints associated with immobile jobs. To stay relaxed, no matter how hard you are concentrating, learn how to sit correctly and preserve the natural curves of your spine. Ask a colleague to give you an occasional neck and shoulder massage when you feel tense. The strokes below relieve cramped muscles and a slumping posture, and alleviate tension in the shoulders and neck which restricts blood flow and causes headaches and eye strain.

IMPROVING POSTURE

■ Choose furniture that helps you to stay comfortable.
■ Use a document holder to keep any papers at eye level.
■ Arrange your desk so that you can reach everything on it without any unnecessary twisting and stretching.
■ Take a short walk during your lunch break to refresh and revitalize body and mind.
■ Organize your work day so that it combines sitting with movement, and stand up every so often to stretch and to move around. This will help to improve your circulation.
■ Make sure you sit on your "sit bones" (where the thighs and buttocks meet) and use a foot stool if your feet do not touch the ground. You can buy a lumbar roll to preserve the back's natural curves. As you sit, think "length, release and width" through the upper body. Keep your elbows by your side, bent at a right angle, and make sure your feet are flat on the floor or the foot stool.

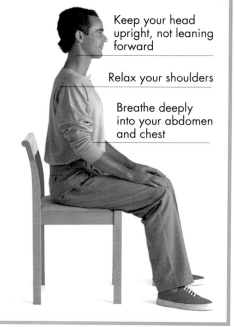

Keep your head upright, not leaning forward

Relax your shoulders

Breathe deeply into your abdomen and chest

EXTENDING UPWARD

This stroke will relieve cramped muscles and slumped posture. Start by placing one hand over your colleague's spine, the other hand over the front of his body. Slowly slide your hands up. As you do so, ask your colleague to lengthen his body upward. Let your front hand stop at his neck, while your back hand continues to glide up over the neck and head. Encourage him to align his neck and head with his spine.

RELAXING TIGHT SHOULDERS

Relieve tension in the shoulders and neck with this stroke. Start by anchoring your fingers over your colleague's shoulders. Then use your thumbs to massage and relax tight and cramped muscles around the upper back, shoulder blades, and the base of the neck. Stroke firmly into these areas, making small circular movements with the pads of your thumbs.

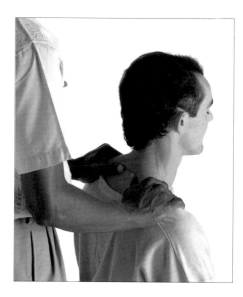

HACKING

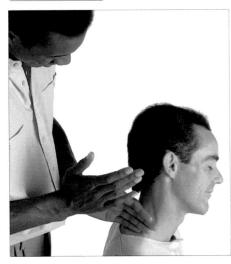

Keep the wrists loose and hands relaxed. Rhythmically drum the sides of your hands over the top of the shoulders, then between the shoulder blades. This relieves headaches and boosts circulation.

LOOSENING THE NECK

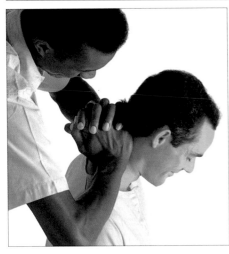

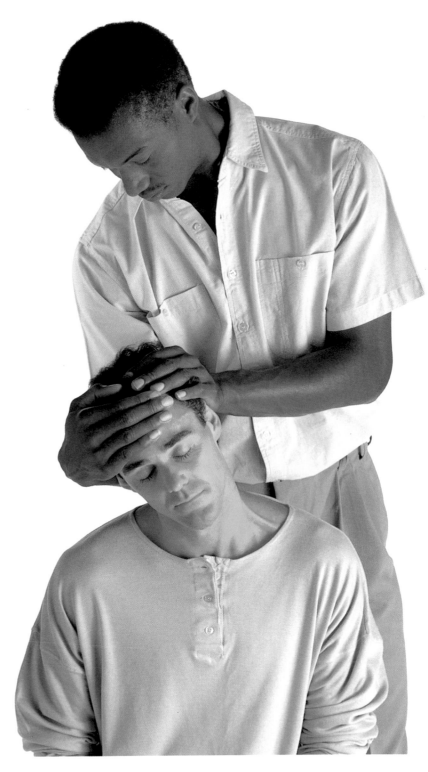

Clasp the fingers together, hands relaxed. Place the heels on either side of the neck just below the skull and, scooping up the muscle, slide them together. Use firm but gentle pressure. Repeat, moving down the neck.

MOVING THE HEAD

This movement releases cramped muscles between the skull and neck, and eases strained eyes. Ask your colleague to let you do all the moving. Gently support the forehead with one hand. With the other hand, roll the head in a circular movement, first to the left, then to the right. Then ask your colleague to lengthen his spine and neck. Ease a tight scalp by working your fingertips up and over the head in small circles, as if shampooing.

SELF-MASSAGE
TO · KEEP · YOUR · BODY · SUPPLE · AND · RELAXED

Simple, quick, and satisfying, self-massage prepares you for the day ahead. It also restores energy and eases tension from a weary body after a stressful, tiring period of work. After a shower, or especially a bath, massaging your body and pampering yourself with lotions and oils is relaxing, keeps your skin in good condition, and boosts your self-esteem. Care for your body using the strokes below and regularly massage the different areas you can comfortably reach. Pay attention to your hands and feet, which are constantly under pressure and strain, and you will find your whole body benefits. To massage and soothe away tension from the face, adapt the strokes on pages 86-87 and 106-107.

MASSAGE STROKES

TAPPING, PUMMELING, AND SQUEEZING strokes can be applied to many different areas of the body to leave you feeling supple and relaxed. The vibration created with tapping strokes revitalizes the body. Pummeling invigorates by boosting blood circulation to the skin and stimulating the nerve endings, and it gives the body a glowing and toned look. Squeezing strokes help restore you after a tiring day by alleviating tension from tight, sore muscles.

TAPPING

This stroke is particularly good in areas where the flesh fits tightly over the bone, such as the scalp, forehead, and upper chest. Keep your wrists loose, elbows at right angles, and tap your fingertips quickly and rhythmically over the area. When working on the scalp, start at the front of the head and move over the back, then down the sides to the neck.

PUMMELING

To break down tension in the shoulders △ and arms, buttocks and thighs, make loose fists and, keeping your elbows and wrists relaxed, drum quickly over the flesh. Let the hand spring away as it touches the skin. Use one hand on the arms, shoulders and neck, two on the lower body.

SQUEEZING

To boost circulation in the thighs and calves, place your hands on the skin, fingers pointing away from you. Press with the thumbs and fingers to scoop up flesh, squeeze gently but firmly, and slowly release.

FOOT MASSAGE

AS WELL AS RELAXING the feet, a foot massage relieves tension in the back. To relax the feet totally, start by soaking them for 20 minutes in herbal bath salts. Close your eyes, breathe deeply and relax your body. Dry each foot by wrapping it in a towel and squeezing all over. Sit on a stool and massage one foot at a time, placing it on your thigh, knee bent up at a right angle. At the end of the massage, briskly rub your feet to revitalize your energy.

1 Squeeze the calves to release stiffness. Rotate the ankle five times in each direction. Stroke around the inside and outside of the ankle bone with thumb and fingers. Hold the foot between both hands for about a minute.

2 Using a firm press-release motion and alternating thumb pads, work rhythmically over the sole. Start at the ridge at the base of the toes, and work to the outside edge of the heel. ◁

Work consistently all over the surface of the sole

Place your foot up on your thigh to massage it

First soak your foot in warm water

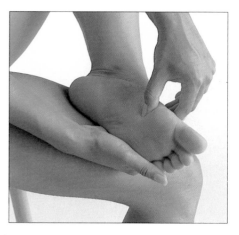

3 Support the foot with one △ hand. With the other thumb pad make tiny circles from the top of the arch to the inner edge of the heel. Repeat three times.

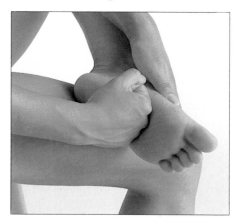

4 Make a loose fist with your right hand and firmly slide your knuckles from the outside edge of the heel to the base of the toes. Repeat this three times. Now gently stretch-pull each toe between thumb and index finger.

HAND MASSAGE

TO KEEP YOUR HANDS supple and free from tension, massage them frequently. This is very important if your work involves many repetitive hand movements, such as pushing, pulling, typing and gripping tools. Use your thumbs, fingers and the heels of your hands to stroke and stretch the muscles and tendons in the hands and wrists. Invigorate your hands at the end of a massage by rubbing them together until vibrant, then consciously relax them.

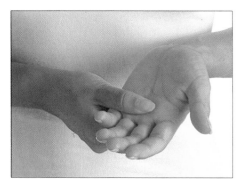

1 Flex your wrist up and down, and turn it from side to side. Then rotate it several times in both directions. To massage your palm, support the back of your hand with your fingers and make small rotary motions with your thumb pad over one spot at a time. Massage the mound at the base of the thumb very well. ◁

2 Start below the lowest knuckle and pull along each finger and thumb with your other thumb and index finger. Press the fingertips. Wiggle finger and thumb joints.

3 Support the hand with your fingers. Slide your thumb down from beside each knuckle to the wrist, between each tendon.

4 Using pressure from your △ thumb pad, squeeze the web between thumb and index finger, making tiny rotary movements on one spot at a time.

LOOSEN THE HANDS

This exercise eases cramped and tight hands. Place your hands together in front of you, palm facing palm, fingers pointing up and elbows at right angles to the body. Slowly raise your elbows so that your palms separate and your fingers press together. ◁

Slowly raise your elbows

Let your fingers press together

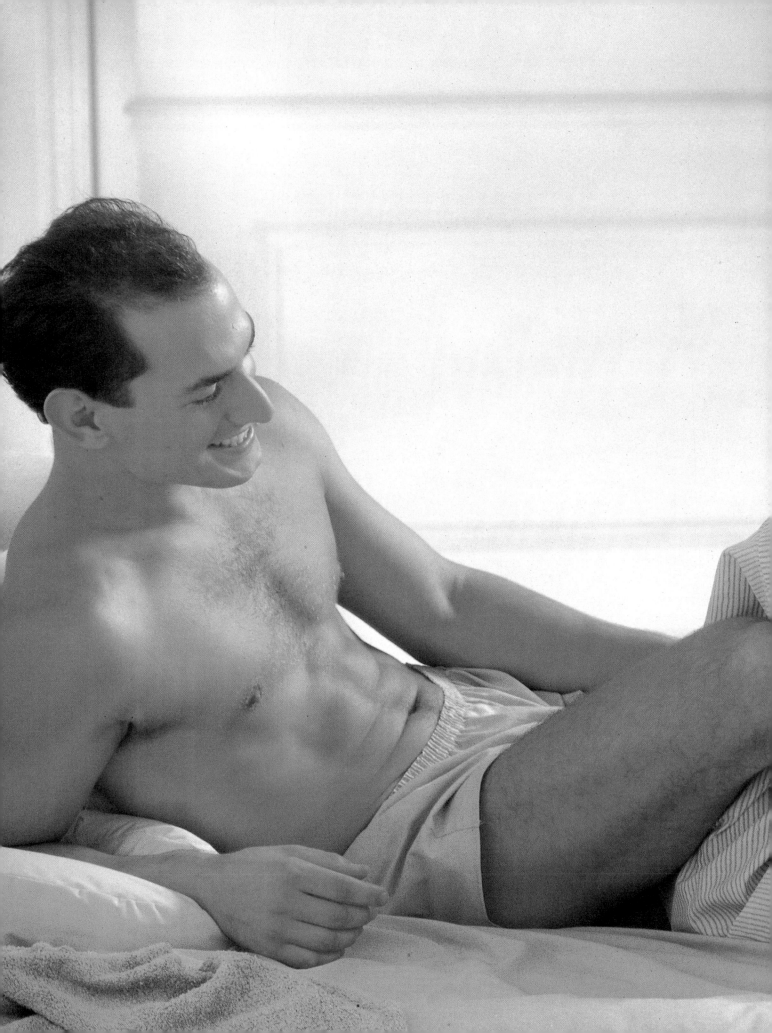

5
RELEASING KEY TENSION AREAS

Certain areas of the body are more prone to the effects of physical and emotional stress. In this section, Nitya Lacroix demonstrates massage sequences to release and relax these tense areas.

FEET & ANKLES
A · MASSAGE · TO · RELAX · THE · WHOLE · BODY

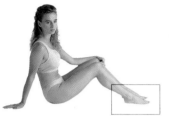

Psychologically as well as physically rewarding, a foot massage dissolves anxiety and stress, eases weariness from an aching body, and stimulates circulation and the nervous system. It can energize the tired, put the insomniac to sleep, and bring relaxation to those who suffer from poor posture. Place your hands over both feet to soothe your partner, then warm and stretch one foot at a time with strokes that ease tension from its bones, tendons and muscle. Revitalize the body by stimulating the thousands of nerve endings on the sole, and loosen the ankle to remove strain from the stance.

MASSAGE TIPS

■ Change your strokes and the pressure of them to suit your partner. Soft strokes increase relaxation; deeper movements revitalize the whole body.
■ The feet are a small area of the body, so use very little massage oil or lotion on them.
■ Raise your partner's knees slightly with a cushion to relax the leg muscles and take tension out of the knees.

WARMING UP THE FEET

Stand by the foot, and place your fingers under it to give support. Alternating hands and applying pressure with your thumbs and then the heels of your hands, make circular strokes toward the sides of the foot. Work up from the base of the toes, over the instep, and toward the ankle. Deepen the pressure on the outward half of each stroke. At the ankle, slide back down the foot and repeat until the foot feels warm, supple and relaxed. ◁

STRETCHING THE FOOT

Place your thumbs and the heels of your hands together over the center of the base of the instep, and press your fingertips into the sole of your friend's foot. With firm pressure, slide slowly out to the sides of the foot. Repeat the stroke several times up over the foot.

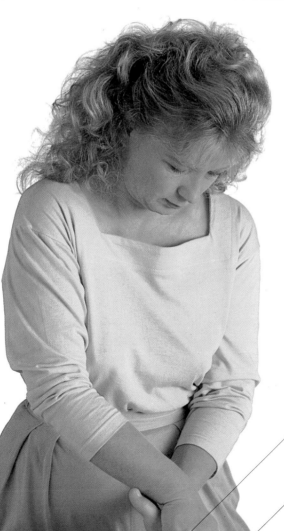

Support the foot with your fingers

Make continuous circles, one hand moving after the other

RELAXING THE TOES

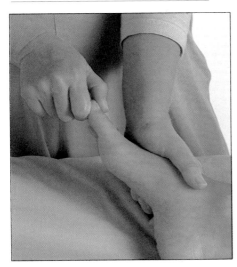

Rotate the toes at the base joint, then wiggle the top joint. Clasp the base of each toe between the thumb and index finger. Stretch along it, then slightly squeeze the tip before pulling out of the toe.

EASING TENSION IN THE ARCH

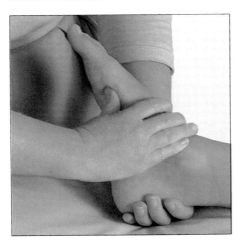

Support the heel with your free hand. Make tiny circles with the tip of your thumb along the arch, working down the inside to the base of the heel. Repeat several times, deepening the pressure.

MASSAGING THE HEEL

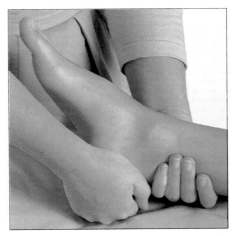

Support the foot with one hand. With the other, make circular strokes over and around the heel with thumb, fingertips and the heel of your hand. Work on one side of the heel, then the other.

KNUCKLE-STRETCHING THE SOLE

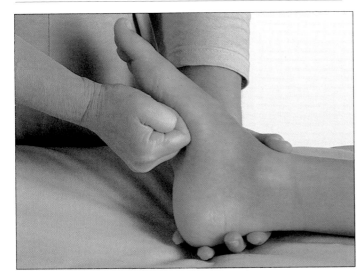

1 Support the foot △ with one hand. Then clench your other hand and draw your knuckles slowly from the heel to the base of the toes.

2 Make tiny circles all over the sole with your thumb tips. Work in strips from the base of the toes to the outside of the heel.

LOOSENING THE ANKLE JOINT

1 Support the ankle △ with one hand. With the other hand, move the foot up and down, holding it at its point of tension. Then release.

2 Turn the foot first to the right, then to the left of the ankle bone. Next, rotate the foot several times in both directions.

LEGS & KNEES
A · MASSAGE · TO · INCREASE · FLEXIBILITY

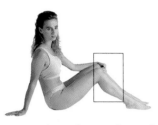

Soft, relaxing massage strokes over the legs will begin to lift strain and tension from the lower half of the body. Use upward-moving strokes to stimulate sluggish blood circulation and help the body to clear itself of toxins. By promoting greater flexibility and movement, the strokes below relax tight tissue and muscle in the key areas of the legs that bear the brunt of muscular tension and postural stress. When strain in the legs is alleviated, the upper half of the body is better able to relax and discharge tension. A good leg massage can renew vitality and ease weariness from a tight, sore back. Combined with a foot massage, strokes on the legs will increase a sense of stability in the body and help your partner to feel more rooted and emotionally secure.

RELAXING THE SHIN BONE

Stand by your friend's lower leg. With your right hand, securely grasp the back of the heel of her foot. Sink the thumb pad on your left hand into the furrow running alongside the outside of the shin bone - do not put pressure on the bone itself. Slowly and steadily move up from the front of the ankle to the outer edge of the knee. At the same time, gently pull the heel of the foot down toward you with your right hand.

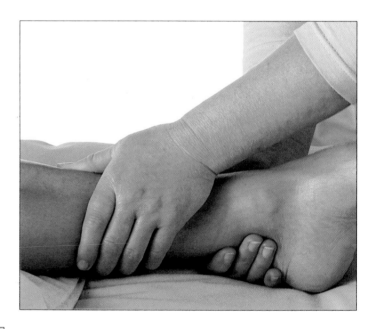

MASSAGE TIPS

■ For this leg massage your partner should be lying on her back. Work first on one leg, then massage the other.
■ Massage the legs with upward-moving strokes.
■ When working on the legs, never put heavy pressure on the bones, particularly the shin and knee cap.

■ If your partner's legs are particularly hairy, you will need to use extra oil or lotion when stroking in an upward direction.
■ Placing a cushion or a pillow beneath your partner's knees keeps them flexed and allows the leg muscles and the lower back to relax.

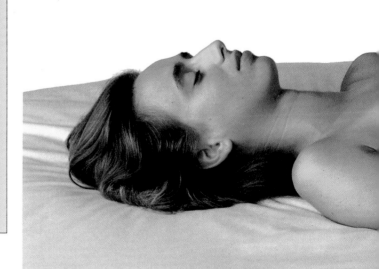

INCREASING FLEXIBILITY IN THE KNEES

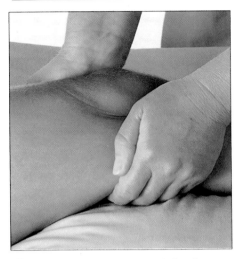

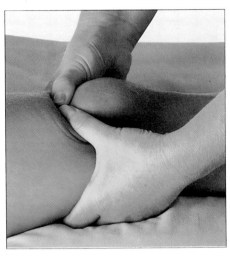

1 Support the back of the knee with your fingers. Thoroughly massage on each side of the knee cap, using the heels of your hands and then the thumbs of both hands. Make continuous circular motions to relax the muscles and ligaments that surround the knee.

2 Still supporting the back of the knee, place your thumbs directly above the knee cap. Add pressure and slowly draw them down around the bone. As the thumbs cross at the base, slip them together up over the knee to the start. Repeat.

DEEP KNEE AND THIGH RELEASE

Place the heel of your left hand immediately above the knee, knuckles slightly flexed. Let your right hand support your wrist and add weight to the stroke. Sink your heel slowly into the tissue and slide it gradually up. Release pressure near the top of the thigh, and slide your hand up and around the hip.

Your free hand supports the wrist

Apply pressure from the heel of your hand

PELVIS & GROIN

A · MOVEMENT · TO · RELEASE · TENSION

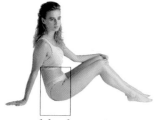

The pelvic area is the site of deep passions and primal responses, such as survival, anger, sexuality, joy and pleasure. If emotional and physical tension build up in this area, they begin to cut us off from these instincts. Touch can restore vitality and help us integrate these emotions. Relax the pelvis with a passive movement that releases tension from the hip and opens up the groin. As the pelvis relaxes correctly, it assures better support for the spine and upper body.

MASSAGE TIPS

■ With your partner lying on her back, stand by her leg.
■ Use this movement after massaging each leg. Work on one side, then the other.
■ Encourage your partner to let you do all the moving, and make sure you are sensitive to her ability to relax.

PELVIS AND HIP RELEASE

1 Support the leg by placing your left hand beneath the knee, your right hand under the heel of the foot. Push up from the heel to bend the leg.

2 Place your left hand over the knee. Move it toward the upper body to stretch the lower back and the buttocks and thigh muscles deeply. ◁

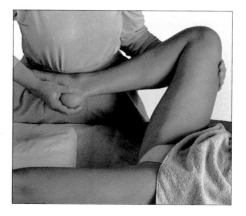

3 Slide your left hand to the △ side of the thigh, and let the leg fall gently into this support.

4 Rock the leg slightly back and forth if you feel a point where it resists any movement.

5 Bring the leg gently back to the starting position and slowly lower it to the mattress.

SHOULDERS & NECK
A · MASSAGE · TO · RELIEVE · CONTRACTION

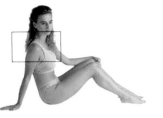

Most people experience a stiff neck and tight, painful shoulders at some time in their lives. Use the massage sequence below to ease tension from this area. By relaxing the chest and releasing the neck away from the shoulders, you bring the neck in line with the spine, helping your partner to regain a more balanced, graceful posture. Once this area starts to relax, massage more deeply along the neck and shoulder muscles, focusing on the often tense area under the ridge of the skull.

> ### MASSAGE TIPS
> ■ Be sensitive with your strokes when you massage the often tight and painful area of the neck. It may be especially tense under the base of the skull.
> ■ To relax both the shoulders and the shoulder blades further, apply the strokes used in *the guard* pages 47-49.

OPENING AND RELAXING STROKE

1 Standing behind your friend's head, let both hands glide down the breastbone, then fan your hands out over the lower rib cage and down both sides of the body.

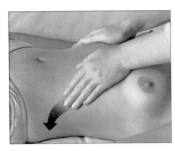

2 Steadily pull up both sides of the ribcage. When you reach the arm-pits, flex your wrists to move your hands back onto the chest.

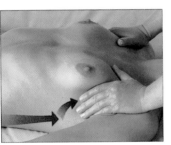

3 Swing your hands out over the shoulders. Draw the heels behind the shoulders to the neck. Your fingers slide along each side of the top of the spine. ▽

4 Pause to let the neck relax. Pull up behind the neck, using pressure from the fingertips. Lift the head slightly at the hairline and steadily draw out of the back of the head. Repeat the movement three times.

NECK AND SHOULDER STRETCH

1 Roll your friend's head into your right hand. Place your left hand sideways over the top of the neck, just below the base of the skull. Steadily glide down the neck so that pressure from the heel of your hand stretches the thick layer of muscle that lies at the side of the neck and behind the shoulder.

Support the head with your right hand

The shoulder gently expands outward under your stroke

Glide firmly down to the shoulder

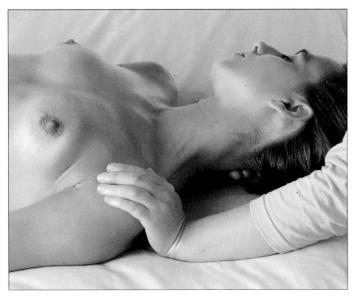

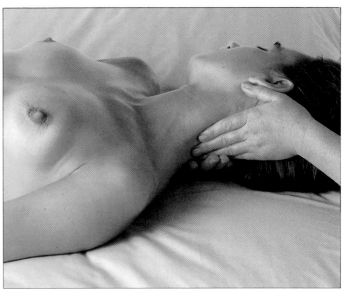

2 Flex your wrist, so that your hand encircles the shoulder joint, and with a lighter touch glide your hand smoothly up behind your friend's shoulder and neck.

3 Continue over the side of the head, stroking your thumb behind the ear. Draw the stroke out through the hair. Repeat the sequence twice, deepening pressure on the first downward motion.

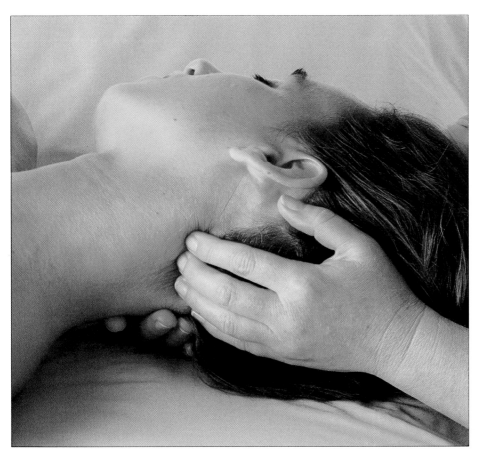

RELAXING THE BASE OF THE SKULL

1 With your friend's head still resting in your right hand, slowly sink your fingertips into the muscle under the base of the skull. Make tiny rotary motions on one spot at a time, moving in deeper as the tissue relaxes. Work gradually to finish just alongside the spine. Be sensitive: this area is often tight and painful. ◁

2 Roll the head into your left hand and repeat the neck and shoulder stretch, followed by the fingertip massage above.

3 Bring the head back in line with the spine. Finally, to integrate all your strokes for a harmonizing effect on the body, repeat the opening movement on page 103.

HEAD & FACE
A · MASSAGE · TO · EASE · AWAY · STRESS

A head and face massage will calm and revitalize your friend by soothing away trapped tension. It can be a wonderful way to begin or end a massage, and it brings great relief and relaxation when combined with strokes on the neck and shoulders (see pages 103-105). This sequence lifts tension caused by worry from the forehead, temples and scalp. It also eases away emotions such as anger, fear, sadness and disappointment locked into the facial muscles. Begin by standing behind your friend's head and take it in your hands, giving her time to relax and become familiar with your touch. You can also use the strokes on pages 86-87 to relax the face.

MASSAGE TIPS
■ The face is an intimate part of the body, and it is important to touch it with great sensitivity and awareness, applying your strokes firmly and steadily.
■ The facial skin is quite oily, so very little, if any, extra lotion is needed on your hands during a head and face massage.
■ Before massaging around the eyes, first ask your partner to remove contact lenses.

FOREHEAD

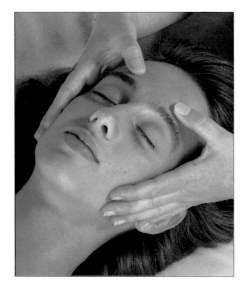

Use this stroke to ease away any anxiety, stress and worry that has gathered around the brow. Place your thumbs over the center of your friend's forehead, just above her eyebrows, gently resting your hands on the head. Steadily draw your thumbs outward. Complete this relaxing stroke by sweeping your hands around the temples. Repeat the stroke, moving up over the entire forehead.

EYEBROWS AND EYES

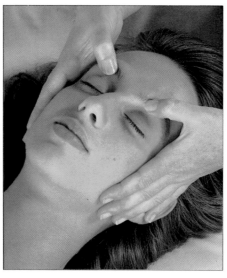

Using a firm pressure, glide your thumbs just under your friend's eyebrows, moving from the inner to the outer edge. Complete this stroke by sweeping out over the temples. Now, using only your fingertips, softly stroke just above, then just below the eyes, always moving your fingertips outward from the eyes.

CHEEKBONES

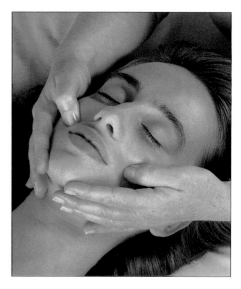

Place your thumb pads on each side of the bridge of the nose and steadily draw them down each side of it, moving out into the muscle just below the cheekbone. Be firm but sensitive in this often tight area, and never put pressure on the cheekbone itself. Take the stroke out to the sides of the face and across the scalp. Complete the movement by sweeping out through your friend's hair.

CHEEKS AND JAW

Bring suppleness to the face with this stroke. Start by making small circles with your fingertips around your friend's mouth and over her cheeks and jaw. Work into the muscles of one area at a time, and focus particularly on the jaw joint.

CHIN AND JAWBONE

1 To relax the mouth, gently push down on the chin using your thumbs. Support the chin from beneath with your index fingers, and then knead it with short thumb strokes. Now gently stroke under the chin, up toward the jaw, with your fingers. ▷

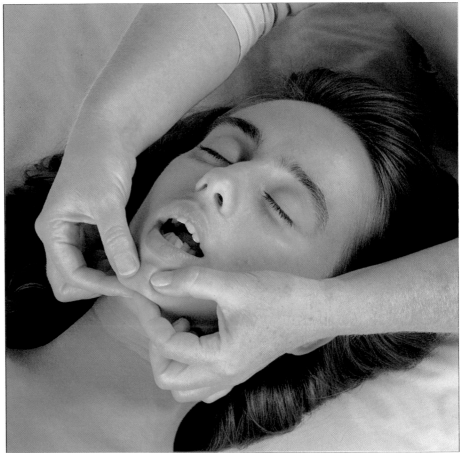

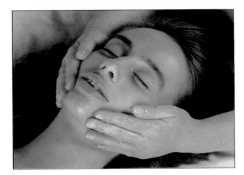

2 Cup your hands over the △ jawbone, fingers meeting at the chin. Help the jaw to relax further by softly drawing your hands up over the jawbone and toward the ears. Draw out across the head and through the hair.

EARS

An ear massage relaxes the whole body. Support the ears with your index fingers. With your thumbs, make tiny circles over the lobes and up along the sides of the ears. Then use your fingertips to stroke around and behind the ears.

SCALP

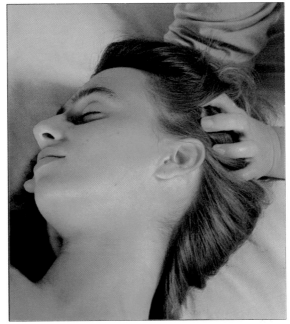

1 Roll your friend's head into your right hand. Make small circles over her scalp with the fingertips of your left hand, as if shampooing. Work thoroughly (quite vigorously) from the base to the top of the skull. Turn the head to work on the right side. ◁

2 Bring the head in line with the spine. Then calm your friend by drawing your hands gently out through her hair in a soothing way.

SPINE & LOWER BACK
A·MASSAGE·TO·LENGTHEN·AND·RELEASE

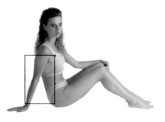

A full back massage, with emphasis on the spine and lower back, greatly eases the effects of stress throughout the body, and enhances physical and psychological well-being. Your smooth, flowing strokes stretch the muscles and tissue, and in so doing, define the shape and contours of the back, and help restore to the spine the relaxation and flexibility essential for easy mobility and whole body health. The stronger strokes along the spinal muscles, and on the sacrum and lower back, bring deep relief to aching and contracted muscles.

MASSAGE TIPS

■ Begin by spreading lotion or oil evenly over the whole back to ensure that your strokes will be smooth and soothing.
■ Do not apply excess oil as this stops your hands gripping or sinking deeply into the muscles.
■ Start with the complete back stroke, which is a pleasurable way to help your partner relax and let go of tension.

COMPLETE BACK STROKE

1 Stand behind your friend's head, hands on the top of her back, fingers pointing downward. Glide firmly down each side of the spine. Fan out over the hips. Pull up the sides of the rib cage. ▷

2 Pull your hands around the shoulder blades, then flex the wrists so that your hands glide around the shoulders. Draw them up the back of the shoulders and neck, and out through the hair. Repeat several times, then feather stroke up the back (see page 121).

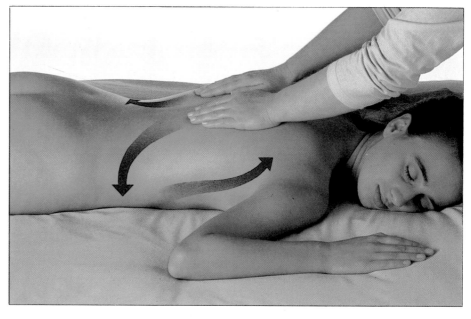

THE SPINE

1 Place your thumbs in the furrows on each side of the top of the spine. Keep your hands on the body. Slowly and steadily slide your thumbs down each side of the spine. Return to the top of the spine by sweeping around and up the sides of the body and over the shoulders. Repeat three times, increasing pressure on each downward stroke.

2 Alternating one thumb with the other, make short, firm strokes down one side of the spine at a time. Work around the sides of the vertebrae, focusing on knotted, tight areas. Then repeat this step down the other side of the spine. ▷

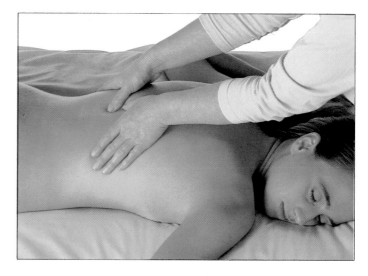

SOOTHE THE SACRUM

Stand by your friend's hip, your thumbs resting on the base of the spine, hands on the buttocks. Massage up and over the sacrum, making small circles with your thumb pads, one following the other. Then, using the whole surface of one hand, softly make circular strokes over the area.

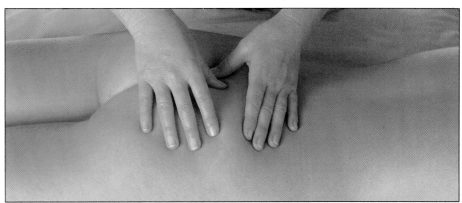

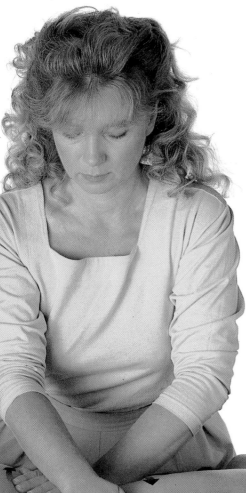

RELAXING THE LOWER BACK

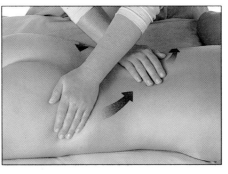

1 Stand beside the back, placing your hands on each side of it, fingers pointing away. Move the hands toward each other.

2 Move your hands diagonally past each other, round the sides of the body, then back to the start, making an unbroken figure of eight movement. ▽

STRETCHING AND RELEASING

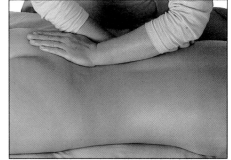

Standing on the left side of the lower back, hook the heel of your right hand into the muscle below the ribs, fingers pointing to the neck. Anchor the heel of your left hand into the lower back, fingers pointing down. Slowly slide your hands in opposite directions, the main pressure and motion in the hand moving down. Release as this hand reaches the buttocks. Repeat on the right side.

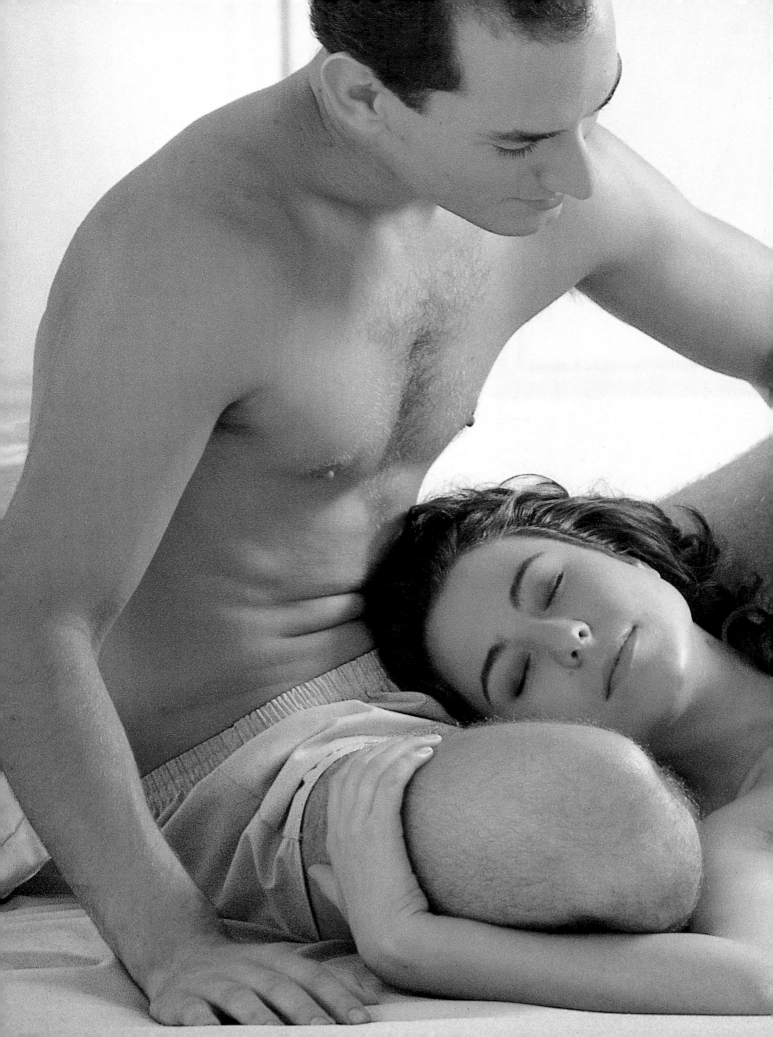

6
EASING
EMOTIONAL
STRESS

Stress can disturb emotional well-being, and
if prolonged it depletes energy and causes
ill-health and anxiety. This section of
the book shows how to calm and refresh the
mind, replenish your resources and ease
emotional tension using massage, breath
awareness, relaxation techniques,
and meditation.

WAYS TO CALM
AND · SOOTHE · THE · BODY · AND · MIND

It is increasingly important today to find ways to relax both the mind and body, and to restore balance to our lives. Soothing and calming an overactive mind, disturbed emotions, or a tense body is possible if we take the time and care to separate ourselves from the whirlwind of activities and demands made upon us in a constantly changing, challenging world. The following suggestions, which include massage techniques, self-help ideas, meditation and relaxation tips, together with body and breath awareness exercises, provide some simple and nourishing ways to regain a sense of harmony, wholeness and equilibrium.

SOOTHING MASSAGE

IN MASSAGE THERE ARE several ways to soothe an anxious or very tense person. Try a full body massage, using mainly smooth, flowing strokes (see *soothing strokes* pages 120-21). This will relax your partner physically and psychologically. Hand stroking gently down the body, especially over the limbs (see page 121), calms by drawing energy away from an overactive mind. A relaxing foot massage eases nervous

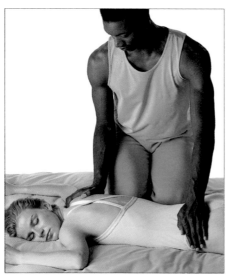

tension and anxiety, and will coax the insomniac into sleep. Harmonious connection holds (see pages 66-69) are restful. They help expand breathing, bring a feeling of integration and balance to the body, and allow your partner time to assimilate and integrate her thoughts and emotions.

The calm, still touch of your hands on the body instills a sense of peace in your partner. ◁

MEDITATION

ONE OF THE SIMPLEST and most effective ways to meditate involves using a breath awareness technique. To meditate in this way, set aside at least twenty minutes every day and find a quiet place to sit. Take a few minutes to relax your body consciously. If possible, sit on a small cushion on the floor, keeping your legs crossed and your back straight. If you find this difficult, sit on a chair that will help you keep a good posture. With practice this meditation will help to quiet your mind and bring you a new awareness of your body. If you feel too anxious or tense just to sit and meditate, then first do some exercise to help you discharge pent-up energy. You will then be able to sit and meditate peacefully.

MEDITATING WITH BREATHING

Close your eyes and focus your whole attention on your breathing. Inhale and exhale through your nose. Let the breath flow gently in and out of your body. Allow it to sink down into your abdomen, and feel the rise and fall of your stomach. Do not force your breathing in any way. Whenever a thought arises in your mind, bring your attention back to your breathing.

BREATHING

BREATHING CAN ALSO BE COMBINED with imagery and with touch, as in the two exercises below, to help you relax both body and mind. The relaxation through breath exercise assists with the loosening of tension and control from the body. The second soothing exercise helps you release the day's stress and anxiety. It will help settle you physically and emotionally, and can induce a relaxing sleep if you are feeling nervous or too mentally active.

RELAXATION THROUGH BREATH

1 Lie on a firm base. Imagine that your weight is sinking down into the ground. As your body becomes heavier, feel the ground receiving your weight.

2 Now focus on and direct your breathing to all parts of your body. Start with your toes and move slowly up to the head. With every exhalation, allow each area to soften and relax. Pay special attention to the legs, pelvis, back, shoulders, arms, neck and head.

3 When your whole body feels relaxed and heavy, focus on the abdomen, then the chest. Feel them expand as you inhale and contract as you exhale. Let your mouth open slightly and your jaw soften. Imagine that the tension in the muscles around your eyes and forehead is melting. Now rest and enjoy complete relaxation, trusting the full support of the ground beneath you.

MELTING AWAY TENSION

Combine touch with breathing to help you let go of tension and anxiety. Lie on your back, either on the floor or on a mat, and let your whole body relax. Then place your right hand over the lower part of your abdomen and your left hand over your heart. Imagine that the warmth and contact of your hands is melting these areas. Let your breathing softly wash through your body. Feel your chest and abdomen as they gently rise and fall beneath your hands. ▽

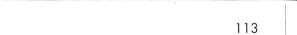

WAYS TO REFRESH
AND · RESTORE · THE · BODY · AND · MIND

When we are healthy, happy, and full of vitality, the body finds a natural balance between activity and relaxation. Sometimes, however, physical and psychological problems make us lose our zest for life: we may drag ourselves half-heartedly through the day, and are unable to find satisfaction in rest. Fatigue, low energy, depression, and a sluggish metabolism prevent us from living fully. By taking care of the needs of the body, mind and spirit, we can restore and replenish ourselves. Then we can move harmoniously from action to inaction and, refreshed and renewed, again take up our activities enthusiastically. The suggestions below help restore and replenish vitality with massage techniques, breathing and movement exercises, sensory awareness meditation, and self-help tips.

REVITALIZING THE BODY

WHEN YOUR VITAL ENERGY is low you may feel unhealthy, inert and heavy, and this only depletes your energy further. The simple self-help techniques below will help reverse this cycle by lifting your spirits and enhancing your bodily and emotional well-being. Use them as part of a daily routine to enliven yourself and boost your self-image.

MASSAGING THE BODY

Turn your morning shower into a refreshing ritual. With a loofah or sponge, rub up over the limbs and torso toward the heart, sloughing away dead cells from the skin and boosting your circulation. Follow a warm shower with a cold one, and be amazed at how invigorated you feel. Smooth and warm your whole body with lotion, and then treat and pamper yourself with a self-massage. Use hacking, tapping and pummeling strokes (see pages 91, 92 and 93). These will increase the blood supply to the skin and stimulate the nervous system. ▷

EATING WELL

Improve your diet by eating plenty of whole foods, fruit and vegetables. Avoid tempting, sticky, sweet foods and artificial stimulants including caffeine, alcohol and nicotine. The boost they give is short-lived, and they rob you of essential energy.

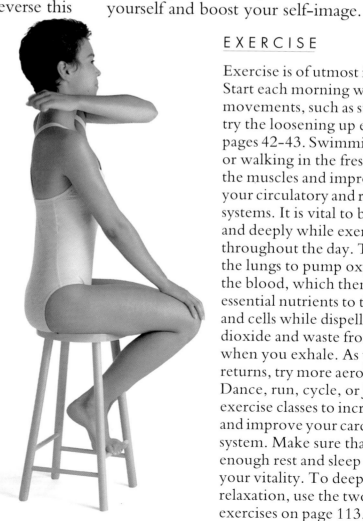

EXERCISE

Exercise is of utmost importance. Start each morning with gentle movements, such as stretching, or try the loosening up exercises on pages 42-43. Swimming regularly or walking in the fresh air tones the muscles and improves both your circulatory and respiratory systems. It is vital to breathe fully and deeply while exercising and throughout the day. This enables the lungs to pump oxygen into the blood, which then supplies essential nutrients to the tissue and cells while dispelling carbon dioxide and waste from the body when you exhale. As your energy returns, try more aerobic exercise. Dance, run, cycle, or join aerobic exercise classes to increase stamina and improve your cardiovascular system. Make sure that you get enough rest and sleep to replenish your vitality. To deepen your relaxation, use the two breathing exercises on page 113.

MASSAGE TO RENEW

WHEN MASSAGING A PARTNER who displays signs of fatigue or low vitality, you should first try to determine what type of massage is needed to nourish and enliven the body and spirit.

RESTFUL MASSAGE

With someone who is exhausted from overwork or lack of sleep, use mostly *effleurage* strokes (see pages 120-21) to nourish, calm, soothe, and provide a much-needed rest to restore energy.

REVIVING MASSAGE

Deeper strokes moving toward the heart revitalize your partner. Stimulating strokes at the end of a massage, such as pummeling and hacking (see pages 93 and 91) and cupping (see page 125), help your partner feel alive and vibrant.

MASSAGE FOR ZEST

If the muscles look undertoned and your partner complains of being sluggish and drained over a period of time, first use relaxing massage strokes. Follow them up with invigorating movements, such as kneading, wringing and deeper tissue work (see pages 124-25). These help to eliminate waste products from the muscles. They also stimulate the blood circulation and nervous system, and increase muscle mobility.

Kneading the chest muscles eases tension and boosts vitality. ▷

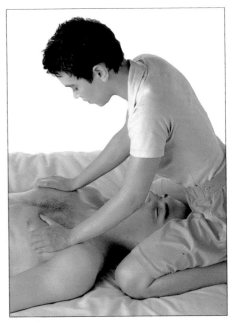

ENHANCING THE SENSES

LOW VITALITY DULLS the senses and decreases your enthusiasm for life. To bring back your sensitivity and joy, and to help you feel more alive, try this sensory awareness meditation to enhance the five senses.

Taste Prepare a varied, delicious and nutritious meal. Eat it slowly, chewing each mouthful up to 40 times before swallowing. Notice the different textures and flavors, and the oral sensations of spiciness and delicacy, sweet and sour.

Touch Begin to explore the many experiences of touch that surround you. Imagine that you are a potter or a sculptor and let your hands mould around the varied shapes of objects. Feel the differences between square and round, soft and hard, delicate and rough, or hot and cold. Touch a friend, an animal, a flower or tree.

Sight Allow your eyes to become receptive. Go into a garden and look at flowers and trees as if you are seeing them for the first time. Take in all the nuances of shape, color, and vibrancy.

Sound Sit quietly with your eyes closed. Then become aware of everything you can hear. Listen to the various noises around you. Distinguish between individual sounds such as people talking, birds singing, and cars passing.

Smell Increase your olfactory senses by focusing your attention on all the scents and odors that surround you. Smell the aroma of food, the perfume of flowers, and the varying fragrances of the countryside and the city.

SENSUAL STROKES
MASSAGE · TO · FREE · SEXUAL · TENSION

To deepen tenderness with your partner, it is important to enjoy a fulfilling sexual relationship. Yet stress, fatigue, and anxiety can all inhibit sexual intimacy and happiness. Suppressed emotions and deep-rooted fears about sexuality, as well as harmful postural habits, can reduce sexual spontaneity and vitality. A loving and sensitive massage is the ideal way to enhance mutual relaxation and intensify sensuality. You can take turns treating each other to a pleasurable full body massage. The following strokes and relaxing exercise will help free sexual energy trapped in the pelvis, buttocks and thighs.

FOCUSING YOUR STROKES

■ Pay special attention during your massage to the diaphragm and abdomen. Strokes on these areas will deepen your partner's breathing and help increase his emotional relaxation (see *the superman* pages 72-77).

■ Devote time to massaging the lower back, buttocks, pelvis and legs. Focus especially on your partner's thighs and groin area.

■ When you are working on the front of the body, particularly with women, focus your strokes on the thighs and the inner leg muscles. Sexual tension is often held in this area of the body, inhibiting sexual happiness.

KNEADING

Ease your partner's back as he lies on his front (see pages 108-109). Then knead the buttocks, thighs and hips. Place both hands on his body, fingers pointing away from you. Press and scoop the flesh between the thumb and fingers of one hand, and release it into the waiting hand. Roll the flesh between the hands.

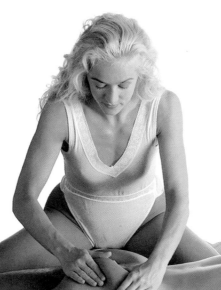

CRADLING THE PELVIS

For further relaxation, slide your left hand under the left side, your right hand under the right side of the pelvic bone. Ask your partner to drop the weight of his pelvis down into your hands, and to breathe deeply into his abdomen.

Cradling the pelvis with your hands is very reassuring

SOOTHING THE THIGHS

1 Lift and release the legs and feet (see page 62). Place your hands parallel, facing in opposite directions, just above the knee, and glide steadily up the thigh.

2 Slide your left hand around the inside of your partner's thigh and groin. Rest it on the inside leg while the right hand continues around the hip. ▷

3 When both hands are parallel on each side of the leg, draw them down behind the leg to the knee, then return to the start of the stroke. Repeat several times.

RELAXING THE INNER THIGH AND GROIN

1 Bend the knee to raise the leg. Let the leg lean out to the side into the support of your arm.

2 Place your hand on the inner leg just above the knee. Add pressure with the heel of your hands and slide up toward the groin. ▷

3 Sweep the edge of your hand and fingers around, into the groin, and back down the leg. Repeat on other parts of the inner thigh.

SELF-HELP · PELVIC ROCK

1 Lie down, knees raised, feet apart. Relax your shoulders and back into the mattress. Your partner places his left hand on your leg, right hand on your abdomen. Inhale deeply as you tip your pelvis back to the mattress.

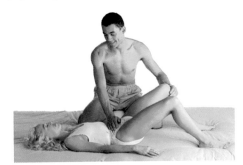

2 Exhale as if releasing down △ through your genitals and tilt your pelvis toward the ceiling.

3 Gently rock your pelvis back and forth in this way, building up to 20 complete movements.

EMOTIONAL TENSION
AND · THE · EFFECTS · OF · MASSAGE

The body, the mind, and the emotions are intrinsically related, and this ensures that what affects one part of us affects the whole. A healthy person constantly moves between action and inaction, tension and relaxation, and it is this ebb and flow that sustains the balance and harmony of the whole person.

We can see this balance in action every day. When we muster and use all our responses to meet a challenge or crisis, healthy, natural tiredness ensues. This allows us to relax, to sink into deep sleep, and vitality is restored. If, however, the cycle of activity and rest is disturbed, we become fatigued and depleted of energy. The subsequent inability to cope makes us ever more distraught. The body of a relaxed, responsive person quickly releases excessive emotions by a natural elimination process. While experiencing sadness, anger or fear, the body trembles and shakes, tears flow, the skin sweats and sounds are emitted, giving expression to the emotions. This, the body's natural releasing process, discharges tension and allows the mind and emotions to return to a poised and stable state. If feelings are constantly suppressed, one's physical and mental health can be damaged. Emotional disorders can result in panic attacks, anxiety, irrational mood changes, and depression. Prolonged stress attacks the body, causing problems ranging from insomnia, ulcers and muscular pain, to hypertension, lethargy, lung and heart problems, and skin diseases.

MASSAGE TO HEAL AND RESTORE

Massage plays a vital part in restoring unity and balance to the body, mind and emotions because it sets in motion the body's own healing process. Touch is vital to our health and happiness, and massage is an excellent medium for its healing qualities. When it is practiced with love and tenderness, and without judgment or criticism, massage is a nonintrusive way to help the body relax and open up. It creates precious time for someone to rest and become refreshed, while receiving physical and emotional care and nourishment. Massage allows us the opportunity to breathe fully, acknowledge the body, and get in touch with underlying emotions, then assimilate them in a gentle and unthreatening way. During massage, the caring touch, the warmth of the hands upon the body, and the reassurance of another person's caring presence remind us that we are not alone.

UNLOCKING EMOTIONAL TENSION WITH MASSAGE

While the techniques of massage are of great importance, it is more essential to develop sensitivity in the hands so that we can feel where and how to touch. Then, even the gentlest placing of hands on the body can dissolve the deepest levels of emotional tension. By resting one hand over the heart or gently stroking under the chin, we can softly unlock the protective tension that surrounds sadness. Our strokes can melt tightness in the shoulders or neck that have become stiffly armored against anger and hurt. By massaging and holding the feet we can help return to the body the energy absorbed by an anxious, overactive mind. When caressing the hands, we can replace feelings of fear and alienation with calmness and tranquillity. Finally, when massaging someone who feels whole and happy, the touch of the hands acknowledges the joy and celebration that are an essential part of a vital, healthy and relaxed body.

7
A
GLOSSARY
OF
STROKES

Massage encompasses many techniques which have different effects on the body and mind. In this section, Nitya Lacroix shows the basic strokes that soothe and relax, those that release tension from muscle and tissue, and strokes that invigorate and revitalize.

SOOTHING STROKES
TO · RELAX · AND · CALM · THE · BODY

Smooth, flowing strokes, called *effleurage* in Swedish massage, enhance relaxation and well-being. Prepare and relax your partner by using *effleurage* before and after more invigorating massage, or use it to integrate other strokes. Keeping the fingers together, use the flat of your hands and mould them to the body to make a continuous motion at a steady speed and rhythm. Increase pressure slightly on the first part of the stroke, and return your hands more lightly. When you start to massage an area, use *effleurage* as a main stroke (shown below on the chest) and follow it with smaller fanlike strokes (shown below on the back).

A MAIN STROKE

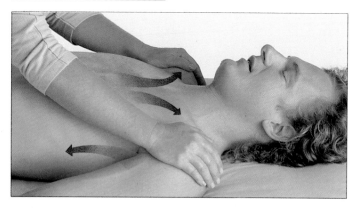

1 Place both hands on the base of the breastbone, fingers pointing to the head. Glide up and fan out over the upper chest toward the shoulders. Let your hands engulf the shoulders, then slide down around the armpit toward the sides of the body.

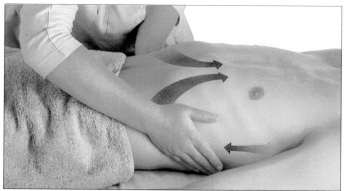

2 Yielding your hands to the body, slide along the side of the rib cage with slightly increased pressure. Return more lightly to the stroke's source. Repeat the sequence three times to induce a deeply relaxing, hypnotic effect on your partner.

FANNING OUT

1 Smaller fan strokes done slowly are relaxing and hypnotic. Performed more quickly, they refresh. Place the flat of the hands on the skin and slide up steadily. After a short distance, fan out to the sides.

2 Glide your hands back down the body, softly shaping them to its contours, then lightly swing your hands back to the source of the stroke. Repeat, taking the stroke higher up the back each time in a flowing, continuous movement. ◁

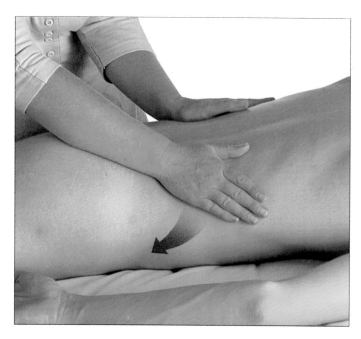

CIRCULAR STROKE

To relax the body before deeper massage, adapt the stroke used on the abdomen in *the superman*, page 74, for the back, sides of the body, and thighs.

CALMING STROKES

STROKING SOFTLY DOWN the body, the flat of one hand following the other, is wonderfully relaxing for your partner. These strokes calm the nervous system and settle the body, while they allow your partner some time to feel and appreciate the full effects of the massage. Calming strokes are particularly beneficial for people who are feeling anxious or stressed, as they direct energy away from an overactive mind back down into the body.

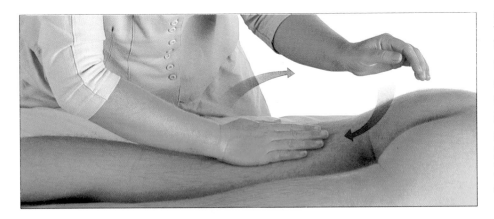

HAND STROKING

Using only the gentlest pressure to caress the skin, stroke slowly downward. Lift the first hand off the body as the other hand starts its downward stroke, and then return it to the body to form a flowing downward movement. Enhance continuity by letting one stroke overlap the other.

FEATHER STROKING

Using the same method as above, let just your fingertips delicately touch the skin in a downward flowing movement. This stroke feels especially good on the arms and legs after a deeper massage.

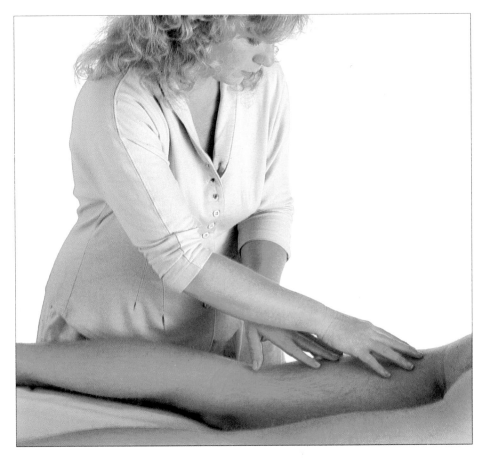

HOW THESE STROKES HELP

■ Soothing strokes are the ideal way to apply oil or lotion to the body and start the massage.
■ They help your partner to get to know his body, and trust and enjoy the contact of your hands on his skin.
■ When applied toward the heart, soothing strokes will boost your partner's blood circulation.
■ Soothing and calming strokes have a euphoric effect and are psychologically beneficial.

RELEASING STROKES
TO · EASE · AWAY · TIGHTNESS · AND · TENSION

Fingers and thumbs are excellent tools in massage for bringing a welcome release of tension to deeper tissue. Before applying releasing strokes, gently soothe your partner with softer strokes, then make sure the skin is fairly free from oil or lotion to enable you to move deeply into the tissue. Apply these strokes with a stronger pressure, but never penetrate the muscles too quickly or sharply. In areas where the muscle forms a thin layer over the bone, use the balls of the fingers and thumbs to press and gently rub the tissue against the bone, helping to eliminate toxic deposits and stimulate the nerve endings.

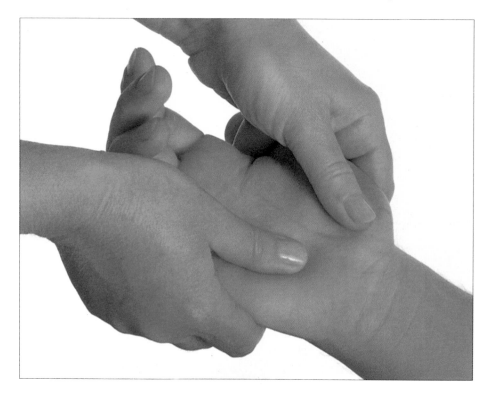

RELEASING THE PALM

Slip your partner's little finger between the last two fingers of your right hand, and his thumb between the last two fingers of your left hand. Rest your fingers on the back of his hand, pressing them upward to stretch and open up his palm. Use your thumbs to work into his palm, making short sliding movements. Then make slow rotary movements with your thumbs over your partner's palm to loosen the muscle and tissue.

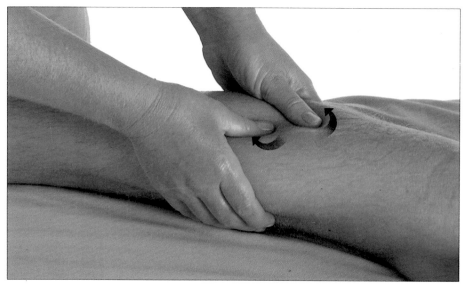

CALF STROKE

This stroke is very effective when used to break down deeply held tension in overworked areas like the calves. Stand by the lower leg with your partner lying down on his front. Then place both hands around the lower leg to support it. Massage into the calf muscles with your thumbs by making continuous circular movements and alternating thumb pads.

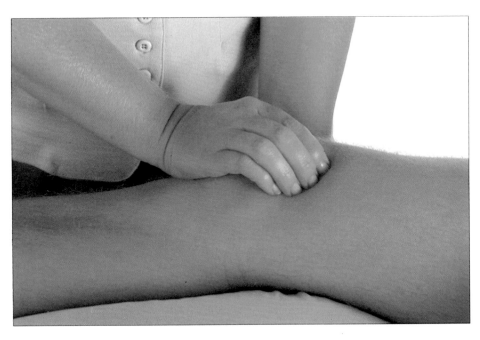

RELAXING THE JOINTS

Use the finger pads to massage all around joints like the elbows, knees, and ankles. Support the area with one hand and with the fingers of your other hand work around the bone, massaging one spot at a time with small circular motions. Do not apply any hard pressure on the bone itself.

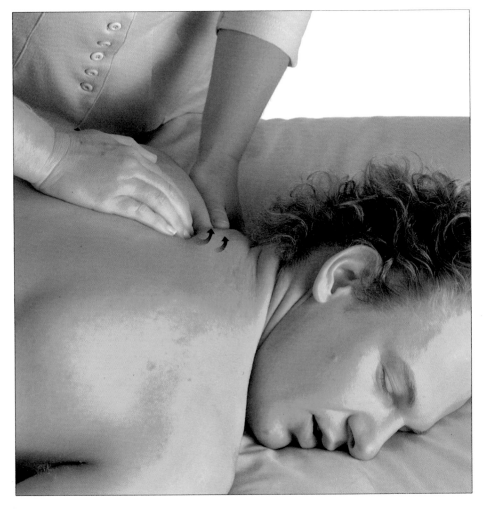

SPIRALING

To free tight muscles and ease tension in the shoulder blades, raise the shoulder slightly with one hand. Place the flat of your other hand on the back, sinking the fingers into the bottom of the area between shoulder blade and spine. Slowly move up, making tiny spirals with your finger pads.

HOW THESE STROKES HELP

■ The dexterous fingers and thumbs can stretch tight muscle and release underlying tension.
■ These strokes release tension particularly well in smaller areas, such as under the skull, around the neck and shoulder blades, and on the calves, hands and feet.
■ When using the pads of the fingers and thumbs, you can work into tense areas close to bone, for example, beneath the skull, along the spine, over the sacrum, around the elbows, knees and ankles.

INVIGORATING STROKES
TO · REFRESH · THE · BODY · AND · BOOST · ENERGY

Kneading and wringing strokes use rolling and squeezing movements to make the muscles feel more pliable and relaxed. Apply these invigorating strokes over fleshy areas such as the buttocks and thighs. They also work well where there is plenty of muscle covering the bone, such as on the shoulders and upper arms. Invigorating strokes are best done when there is little oil left on the body so the hands can maintain a good grip on the flesh.

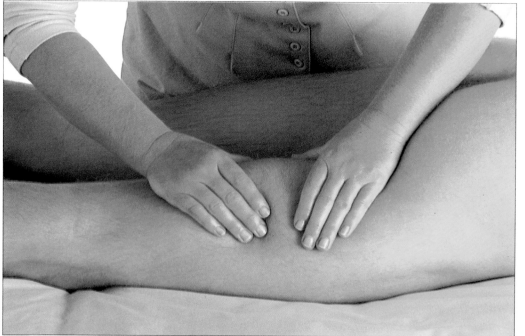

KNEADING

Place both hands on the body, fingers pointing away from you. Press down with one hand to gather and lift the flesh between your fingers and your thumb. Then roll and release it into your other hand. Move the flesh continuously between both hands.

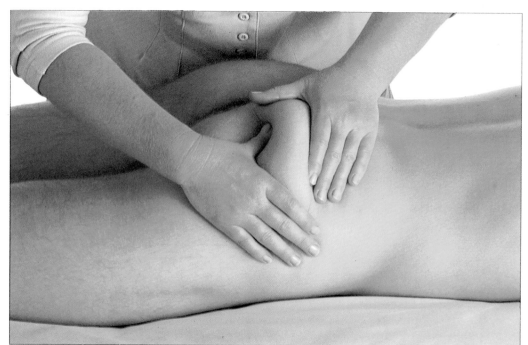

WRINGING

Keep your hands in the same position on the body as in kneading. To create a wringing effect that squeezes even more deeply on the muscle, press deeper with your fingers, and add a little twist into the stroke.

STIMULATING STROKES

BY INCREASING THE BLOOD SUPPLY to the skin, these strokes leave a healthy glow and enliven your partner. They also improve muscle tone. Stimulating strokes are most appropriate for fleshy areas such as the thighs, shoulders and buttocks; do not apply them on bony areas. Use these strokes to revitalize and refresh your partner after a massage, but never introduce them too abruptly, if your partner has fallen asleep, or if he is in a sensitive state. The strokes work well when your partner is sitting or lying. You can make them with the sides of your hands (see hacking, page 91), fingertips, or loose fists (see tapping and pummeling, pages 92-93). Quick, light movements that spring back off the skin are the most effective.

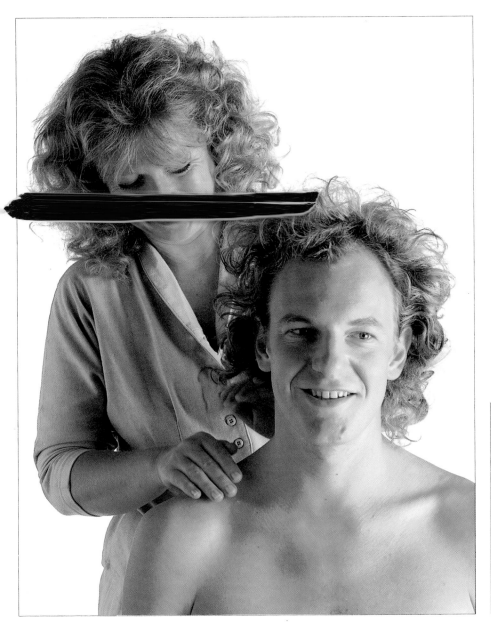

CUPPING

Cupping is used to revitalize low energy levels as it can stimulate both the circulation and the nerve endings, leaving the body feeling alive and invigorated. Cup your hands, keeping your fingers straight and your thumbs pulled in close. The center of your hands will act as a vacuum, sucking up air and drawing the blood supply to the surface of the skin. Now alternating hands, lightly strike your partner's skin quickly and rhythmically. This should make a sound like the tapping of horses' hooves.

HOW THESE STROKES HELP

■ The overall effect of all these strokes is very refreshing.
■ Invigorating strokes help break down both fat deposits and waste products in the tissue. They also increase muscle flexibility.
■ Stimulating strokes will bring suppleness to tense, stiff muscles, while they improve the tone of slack muscles.

INDEX

meditation, 36, 112
mind: calming, 112-13
    emotional stress, 110-18
    refreshing, 114-15

N

neck: balance, 67, 69
    kneading base of, 86
    loosening, 91
    releasing, 42
    relieving contraction,
        103-5
    roots and wings
        massage, 40
    sitting posture, 90
    stretching, 58-9, 104-5
    tension, 13
nervous system, 8

O P

oils, 32, 34
palm of hand, releasing, 122
palpitation, 78
pelvis: balance, 51
    cradling, 116
    loosening up, 43
    pelvic rock, 117
    relaxing joints, 61
    roots and wings
        massage, 41
    tension, 12-13, 102
personality, 14
physical stress, 88-9
pillows, 32-3
posture techniques, 38-41,
    50-3
posture, 14, 90
pressure points, eyebrows,
    87
pummeling, 92, 93, 114

R

refreshing body and mind,
    114-15
Reich, Wilhelm, 9, 128
relaxing hold, 72
releasing strokes, 66, 122-3

restful massage, 115
revitalizing the body, 114
reviving massage, 115
rib cage, 41, 76-7
rocking shoulders, 47
roots and wings posture
    techniques, 38-41
roots and wings massage,
    40-1

S

sacrum, 69, 109
scalp, easing tightness, 91,
    107
sedentary stress, 90-1
self-massage, 92-5
senses, enhancing, 115
sensual massage, 116-17
sexual tension, 116-17
sexuality, 6-7
shaking, ankles, 82
shin bone, relaxing, 100
shoulders: balance, 68, 69
    loosening up, 42
    relaxing joints, 47, 60-1
    relaxing shoulder
        blades, 49
    releasing, 52
    relieving contraction,
        103-5
    rocking, 47
    roots and wings
        massage, 40-1
    self-massage, 93
    sitting posture, 90
    stretching, 48, 104-5
    tension, 12-13, 90
sitting posture, 90
skull see head
sleep, 118
sole of foot, 99
soothing strokes, 112, 120
spine, extending, 48, 52,
    54-5, 108-9
    releasing, 89, 108-9
    roots and wings
        massage, 40
see also back
spiraling, 123
squeezing strokes, 92, 93

stimulating strokes, 125
stoic body type, 16
    profile, 28-9
    program, 78-83
stress, 7-8
    breathing and, 36
    emotional stress, 9,
        110-18
    work-related, 84-95
    your body and, 14
see also tension
stretches: ankle tendon, 83
    back, 79, 109
    buttock, 80
    calf, 81
    neck, 58-9, 104-5
    shoulder, 48, 104-5
    spine, 48
    thigh, 81
strokes: calming, 121
    circular, 74, 120
    complete back, 108
    cross-over, 73
    cupping, 125
    deeper, 35, 80-1
    effleurage, 115, 120
    feather, 121
    hacking, 91, 114
    hand stroking, 121
    invigorating, 124
    kneading, 78, 86, 115,
        116, 124
    pummeling, 92, 93,
        114
    releasing, 66, 122-3
    rhythm and
        sequence, 34-5
    soothing, 120
    spiraling, 123
    squeezing, 92, 93
    stimulating, 125
    tapping, 92, 114
    wringing, 115, 124
superman body type, 16
    profile, 26-7
    program, 72-7
Swedish massage, 120

T

tables, massage, 33
tapping, 92, 114
temples, relaxing, 87
tendons, ankle, 83
tension, 8
    body profiles, 10-29
    massaging tension
        areas, 50, 66
    releasing key tension
        areas, 96-109
see also stress
thighs: deep release, 101
    long stretch, 81
    relaxing, 117
    self-massage, 93
    soothing, 117
    squeezing, 81
thumbs, massaging with,
    74, 122
toes, relaxing, 99
torso: extending upward,
    52
    massage, 50
    roots and wings
        massage, 40
    healing and, 118
    importance of, 6-7, 32
towels, 32

V

verbal instructions, 35, 40
victim body type, 16
    profile, 20-1
    program, 50-5
visualization techniques,
    38-41, 50-3

W

warming up, feet, 98
warrior body type, 16
    profile, 22-3
    program, 58-65
wings, roots and, posture
    techniques, 38-41
work-related stress, 84-95
wringing, 115, 124
wrists, flexing, 65

ACKNOWLEDGMENTS
AND · BIBLIOGRAPHY

AUTHOR'S ACKNOWLEDGMENTS

I would like to thank Sudhir Anna Borowyj who helped me devise the massages; Martin Gerrish for generously lending so much reading material; Anne Geraghty for her constant support; and the Dorling Kindersley team, especially Tina, Susannah, Tim, Barney, and Jenny.

Dorling Kindersley would like to thank Karen Ward for design help; Laura Harper for editorial help; Hilary Bird for the index; Rosalind Priestley for production; Barnabas Kindersley for assisting Tim Ridley; Paul Derrick for assisting Peter Waldman; Trevor Hill for the artwork; O'Connor Dowse for the re-touching; Lilywhites; and all our models: Anneli Adolfsson, Lisa Beer, Lucy Berridge, Anna Borowyj, Tracey Butcher, Claudia Freund, Tushir Jones, Gary Kitchener, Deval Knight, Sarah Lloyd, Ferida Loh, Susannah Marriott, Donnachadh McCarthy, Christian Meyer, Louise Norster, Frank Terry, Tina Vaughan, Mark West, Henderson Williams.

PHOTOGRAPHY

All photography by Tim Ridley except: pages 2-3, 7, 30-31, 37, 44-45, 56-57, 70-71, 84-85, 96-97, 110-11, 119, 128 by Peter Waldman; front jacket by Steve Gorton.

MAKE-UP AND HAIR

Jenny Jordan, with make-up by Chanel; except pages 1, 12-13, 22-25, 38-39, 58-69, 92-95, 112 by Bettina Graham.

BIBLIOGRAPHY

Many great pioneers have laid the foundations that link psychology, the emotions and bodywork. The lineage begins with Sigmund Freud and progresses with, among notable others, Wilhelm Reich (Character Analysis), Alexander Lowen (Bioenergetics), Ron Kurtz (Hakomi Therapy), Ida Rolf (Rolfing). Influences on re-education of movement and breath awareness for relaxation include F. Matthias Alexander (The Alexander Technique), Moshe Feldenkrais (The Feldenkrais Method), Judith Aston (Patterning). Recommended reading: *Character Analysis*, W. Reich; *The Language of the Body*, *Bioenergetics*, A. Lowen; *The Body Reveals*, R. Kurtz & H. Prestera; *Bodymind*, K. Dychtwald; *Rolfing: The Integration of Human Structures*, I. Rolf; *Movement Through Awareness*, M. Feldenkrais; *The Resurrection of the Body*, F. M. Alexander; *The Complete Book of Massage*, C. Maxwell-Hudson.

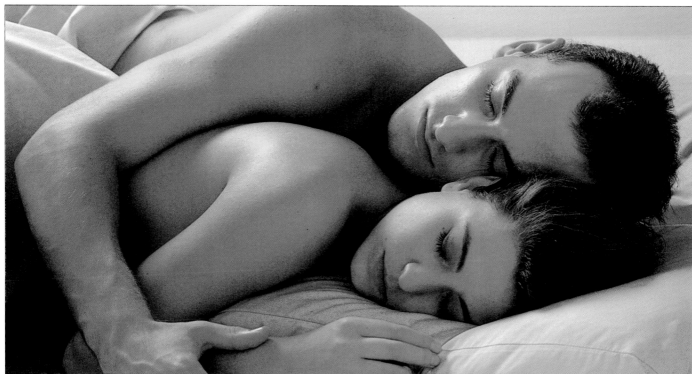